BABY ECOLOGY

Using Science and Intuition to Create
the Best Feeding, Sleep, and Play
Environment for Your Unique Baby

ANYA DUNHAM, PhD

Baby Ecology: Using Science and Intuition to Create the Best Feeding, Sleep, and Play Environment for Your Unique Baby
©2022, Anya Dunham, PhD. All rights reserved.
Published by Encradled Press, British Columbia, CANADA

ISBN 978-1-7778044-0-4 (paperback)
ISBN 978-1-7778044-1-1 (eBook)

Publisher's Cataloging-In-Publication Data
(Prepared by The Donohue Group, Inc.)

Names: Dunham, A., author.

Title: Baby ecology : using science and intuition to create the best feeding, sleep, and play environment for your unique baby / Anya Dunham, PhD.
Description: British Columbia, Canada : Encradled Press, [2022] | Includes bibliographical references and index.

Identifiers: ISBN 9781777804404 (paperback) | ISBN 9781777804411 (ebook)

Subjects: LCSH: Infants--Care. | Human ecology.

Classification: LCC RJ61 .D86 2022 (print) | LCC RJ61 (ebook) | DDC 649.122--dc23

Indexing by Under the Oaks Indexing

Publishing services provided by AuthorImprints.com

For the most amazing humans—our babies—
and for those who grow babies under, or in, their hearts

Ecology: a branch of biology that studies how living things relate to one another and interact with their environment.

Despite technological progress, *baby ecology*—what our babies need from the physical spaces they live in, the care they receive, and their interactions with people in their life—has remained constant and is universal.

CONTENTS

ABOUT THIS BOOK

LOOKING AT BABIES IN A DIFFERENT WAY

When I think back to my first year as a mom, I remember feeling love beyond any experience I had yet had. I was swept off my feet by my fierce need to nurture and protect our baby daughter, by her uniqueness and completeness… but also by worry and doubt. I was ready for the sleepless nights, but not for how heavy the responsibility for a tiny person would feel. I wanted to become the best parent I could be. I read dozens of parenting books and browsed through countless online resources, but found myself in a sea of parenting trends promoting conflicting approaches to every aspect of baby care.

By the time my daughter was born I had a doctorate degree in biology and had spent twelve years doing biological research. So I went to the original sources of knowledge about babies: the scientific studies. I carefully read over eight hundred peer-reviewed publications on infant development, sleep, and feeding, and separated well-substantiated results from preliminary findings and speculations.

I found that science has accumulated a vast amount of knowledge on child development and the ways babies are raised around the world. Different cultures use different approaches they consider natural, and each family creates its own set of unique baby care practices. Imagine these *family practices* as dots; some are quite far apart and some are closer together, but none are exactly the same:

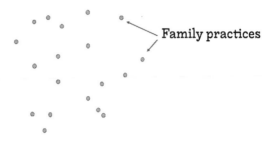

I also realized why there are so many conflicting approaches to baby care. Most scientific studies are designed to answer very specific questions in very specific settings. Their findings are not supposed to be applied beyond a particular situation or stage of development. Yet, sometimes scientific findings get misinterpreted in the media and then amplified by parenting trendsetters who take away select messages that fit their particular philosophy. They create strict parenting "dos" and "don'ts" that presume there is only one correct way. They offer parenting techniques aimed at a particular stage or challenge that often contradict what other experts promote in their own strict guidelines: "sleep train at five months" but "never leave your baby to cry"; "start with purees" but "skip purees entirely"; "always babywear" but "do not restrict free movement." Many techniques come with a sense of pressure: "Do this… or else your baby will not thrive."

The problem is, no parenting trend works perfectly for everyone. Parents who choose to carefully follow one particular trend often discover that not all the recommended techniques work for their baby and family. If we add *parenting trends* to our map of family practices, they would look like this; some work for some families, but none work for all:

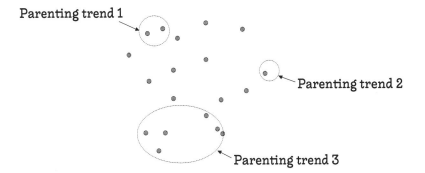

But what if we shift our perspective? What if we saw raising a baby not as a series of parenting techniques, but as an opportunity to nurture a whole person? What if we look at it from the babies' perspective? What do babies really, truly need?

With this new frame of mind, I returned to the research, but this time went a step further. My scientific expertise is in ecology, a branch of biology that studies how living organisms relate to one another and interact with their environments. More specifically, I study habitats: spaces and environments that support life. And so I began to think about baby-care questions from an ecological perspective. Each baby has fundamental abilities and needs universal to all human babies, as well as his own unique traits. His environment consists of the physical spaces he lives in, the care he receives, and his interactions with the people in his life: everything that shapes his day-to-day experiences. In developmental psychology this immediate environment is called the microsystem.[1,2]

I critically examined the scientific studies once again, but this time through the lens of ecology: *baby* ecology. I set out to find answers to these questions:

- What are the fundamental, universal needs of *all* human babies?
- What elements in babies' environment help meet these needs?
- What circumstances make meeting these needs difficult?

After I analyzed the scientific research from this new angle, it became very clear that there will never be one perfect parenting trend; there is not just one "right" way to raise a baby. However, there is a biologically optimal *range* that supports every baby's unfolding natural abilities. This range is the *Optimal Nurturing Environment*, or "the ONE" for short.

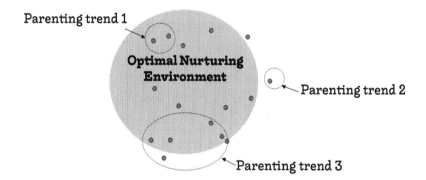

The ONE is based on human biology and is universal: it is the same for all human babies. But it's easy to find yourself outside its range. As shown in the picture above, some family practices fall within the ONE, but others do not; parenting trends sometimes straddle or even fall completely outside it.

Fortunately, there are many ways to create your unique family practices within the ONE. This book will help you find your way.

THE ONE: WHERE NURTURE WORKS WITH NATURE

What is, or will soon be, at the heart of all decisions you make for your baby?

I think I know the answer: love. Love is the foundation.

Building up from love, in the coming chapters I will explore the *universal elements* of a nurturing environment, in each of the major aspects of raising babies: sleep, feeding, and care and play. These are elements that are important for all families to create, regardless of their cultural backgrounds or parenting philosophies and the specific care practices they choose. They matter for all babies. They are the building blocks that we place on the foundation of love to create a nurturing environment, a strong base for baby to grow.

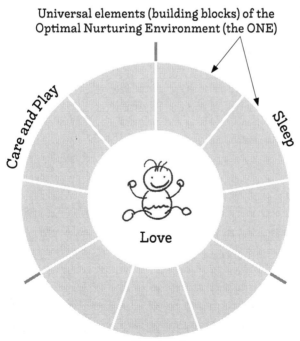

Universal elements (building blocks) of the Optimal Nurturing Environment (the ONE)

We, parents and caregivers, have the extraordinary power to create and protect our baby's environment, especially in the first year. Each baby's development is a result of a dynamic interplay between nature and nurture. If we make thoughtful and intentional choices, we can nurture *with* nature as opposed to working against it. A wholesome, balanced environment gives babies the support and freedom to explore, connect, and express who they are and what they need. It's like a good garden that can support all kinds of unique plants with different traits and strengths.[3] Such an environment has effects that can last a lifetime. It helps biological rhythms emerge and natural development unfold. It supports babies in growing at their own pace and developing their full potential, being the people they are meant to be.

In contrast, when important elements are missing or out of balance, it makes it harder to see who our babies truly are and more difficult to interpret what they are telling us. For example, a baby who has high sleep needs but is chronically tired may appear unsettled and very active, making you think he no longer needs daytime naps; a baby who's been offered solid foods before she was ready may seem like a picky eater. Missing these elements makes it difficult for us to connect with our babies and creates and reinforces patterns that can be hard to change later on.

Some expecting parents plan to rely solely on their instincts. But parenting skills and knowledge don't show up magically once our babies are born. When you become a parent you will feel the power of the caregiving drive. This drive will inspire a fierce desire to protect and nurture your baby—but you won't naturally know how to translate this desire into action, and that's okay. You need the time and space to learn. Two resources you can draw from are scientific knowledge and your intuition. Science can help you with both: it will give you the evidence and a way to separate true intuitive knowledge from biases and fads (more on this in Chapter 5). The ONE approach will help you use the scientific knowledge and your intuition as you care for your baby in ways that match your values and your baby's unique personality, creating a strong nurturing foundation.

As you read about the scientific findings, keep in mind a couple of caveats. First, some aspects of physiology and health have not been studied yet or cannot be studied at all because doing so would be unethical or impossible. For example, finding a threshold for adequate nutrition experimentally by randomly assigning babies to "wholesome diet" and "poor diet" groups is, thankfully, never going to be an option. In such cases the broad picture comes from a patchwork of studies with unavoidable gaps. Second, as Dr. Alice Callahan says in her book *The Science of Mom*, we can't raise the same baby several times in different conditions and note the differences, so science has to zoom out to look at many babies and families to reveal patterns and averages.[4] Knowing such averages—ages, weights, number of feedings, or hours of sleep—can be very helpful, but it's also important to remember that a baby who is truly average in every way exists only in the world of statistics, not in real life. As I walk you through the science on each topic, I will point out cases where science gives us comprehensive answers, where it gives us more of a guidepost or two, and where the true answer will likely never be found (which is sometimes just as important to know).

HOW THIS BOOK IS STRUCTURED

Chapter 1 will give you a sense of what newborns are like and help you prepare your home—and your mind—for your new arrival. Chapters 2 through 4 cover the major topics of sleep, feeding, and care and play during your baby's first year. Chapter 5 will offer you ideas on how to feel more confident and supported on your parenting journey.

Each chapter is divided into two parts. In Part I, I integrate and crystallize the scientific knowledge on each topic. All of the studies I describe are fully referenced, with scientific publications listed at the end of the book. In essence, Part I is about *all human babies* and what science can tell us about their needs.

In Part II of each chapter I offer advice on how to create the Optimal Nurturing Environment – the ONE – *for your unique baby*. First, I use my research training to translate the science into universal elements, the building blocks for the ONE. You will need these building blocks regardless of the specific practices you choose: whether you bed-share or your baby sleeps alone, whether you formula-feed or breastfeed, or whether you choose purees or baby-led weaning. There will be no parenting wars, I promise. Next, I use my perspective as a parent to offer you a stage-by-stage guide, explaining how to put these building blocks into place and what to focus on during various stages of your baby's development. I bring in stories from different families, including my own, describing some of the challenges and joys you may encounter along the way. I invite you to see and understand babies, to think more deeply about them, and to marvel and wonder as you watch your baby grow.

Throughout the book, you will come across the following symbols:

 From Your Baby's Perspective:

Metaphors to help you imagine what our world might look like from your baby's point of view.

**What You
Will Need:**

Suggestions for items to purchase, borrow, make, or prepare as you create a supportive environment for your baby.

**Practical
Tips:**

Ideas on how to make things easier and more enjoyable.

This book is for all babies; I switch between "he" and "she" throughout. Similarly, this book is for all adults who love babies and care for them: when I use "you," it refers to moms or dads (sections on breastfeeding being the only exception). I live in Canada and was fortunate to stay home with my babies for a full year, but I am conscious of the fact that not all families have this opportunity or choose this option. Much of the advice in this book can be used by extended family members or professional daytime caregivers.

· · · · ·

This book merges my scientific training and my own experience of the intense and beautiful early parenting months. I wrote it to guide and support you in nurturing your baby. I hope it helps you see more, understand better, and worry less.

CHAPTER 1
BRINGING YOUR BABY HOME

We are driving from the hospital, bringing our newborn home for the first time. How can this city look the same? How can things remain in their former shapes and places when my whole world has changed? We are home. I am gently holding my baby as she sleeps, the seven delicate pounds, but I feel like I'm holding her life, her future, our future... Jason and I look at each other. The journey has begun, and we're in charge.

Having a baby can feel like a leap into the unknown. No matter how long you have been waiting for this baby, you might be feeling unprepared for the big arrival, and that is perfectly okay. Your baby's needs will be all-consuming but simple: eating, sleeping, exploring, and being cared for in a loving and calm environment. Most of all, your baby will need you: your love, knowledge, attention, and time as you grow and learn together.

In this chapter I have gathered some key concepts to help you prepare for your new arrival. These concepts will also lay the groundwork for the chapters on sleep, feeding, and care and play that follow.

PART I
NEWBORNS: THE SCIENCE

"The child is not an incomplete adult"
                    —Joseph Chilton Pearce, *Magical Child*

O ur babies are a complex mix of competence and needs; they are already complete and still full of potential. It is easy to over- and under-estimate them all at once. For example, we might ask too much of babies logistically, making them conform to schedules or stay up late. On the other hand, we might under-estimate or even miss the amazing things babies can do as we look out for specific milestones. Science tells us that newborns come into the world capable and aware, sensitive, and ready to connect and learn.

Capable and aware

Fifty years ago young babies were seen as blank slates. Scientists were discouraged from studying "passive," "unfinished," and "not yet interesting" newborns.[5,6] Thankfully, many scientific studies have been conducted since, and now we know that newborns are competent from the start. They are not yet mobile or independent, of course: they can't walk like newborn fawns or navigate on their own like newly hatched turtles. The human brain is uniquely capable of complex reasoning and social interactions and, because of that, it takes a long time to develop. This requires humans to have a uniquely long, protected childhood. And our babies come into the world perfectly prepared for just that: growing, connecting, and learning while being fully protected and nurtured by adults.[5]

What Newborns Can Do

Babies develop the ability to hear sounds during the second trimester of pregnancy. In the third trimester a baby can recognize his mother's voice,[7-9] the sound of his mother's native language,[10] and familiar stories she has been reciting.[11] This means babies not only hear quite well, but also pay attention, learn, and memorize even before they are born![8]

Newborns' vision is not fully developed, but they are able to work out the shapes and features of objects that are close to them and that interact with them.[12] Newborns prefer looking at human faces[13] and learn to recognize their mother's face within hours of birth if they are also able to hear her voice.[14] This means that a newborn's vision and ability to recognize patterns are already sufficient to connect the voice she remembers to the face she now sees. Babies learn incredibly quickly!

Newborns can tell if someone is looking at them or away from them.[15] They are calmed by soothing touch, but find it stressful when touched in silence and without eye contact.[16] They are already perceptive.

Babies experience a variety of tastes while still in the womb and right after birth. Amniotic fluid and breastmilk carry flavours from the mother's diet, so baby begins learning about the foods that are important to her family and culture right from the start.[17, 18]

Babies are born with an innate ability to feed well. When a healthy newborn is placed skin-to-skin on his mother's chest after birth and given time, he will use his arms and legs to move to the breast and latch to feed for the first time—remarkably, all by himself.[19] This phenomenon is known as the breast crawl.

Newborns have other innate abilities that are highly complex. For example, when held and supported upright, they might show a coordinated "stepping" movement. This ability lays the foundation for walking as baby gradually gains strength and balance during the first year.[5]

Sensitive

Being tuned into their environment helps babies learn rapidly. At the same time it makes them sensitive and easily overwhelmed, especially in the early weeks. The first twelve weeks after birth are often called "the fourth trimester." During this important transitional period babies are adjusting to life outside the womb and parents are adjusting to their new roles.

 From Your Baby's Perspective:

Imagine how it feels for a baby to be born. She was cozy and snug, connected to a constant supply of nutrients. Her world was stable in its warmth, soft light, gentle motion, and the steady rhythm of a heartbeat. Now the world is big and constantly changing: quiet and noisy, bright and dark, slow and fast, warm and cold... full of unfamiliar sensations, smells, and sights. No wonder babies are most content nestled on a parent's chest in a quiet and cozy space, feeding frequently.

Newborns work hard on adjusting their inner rhythms and states to their environment.[20] Older children and adults are synchronized to the day-night cycle by the biological clocks that control their sleep, alertness, and hunger. These biological clocks are quite stable and slow to adjust to shifts. Think of a time you experienced jetlag; that was your biological clock taking its time to adjust to the new time zone. As you will see in Chapter 2, newborns' biological clocks are not running smoothly yet, and so their physiological processes and rhythms are not yet organized or coordinated. Because of this, maintaining a steady, balanced state is not easy for babies.[21] They are working hard at staying calm and regulated so they can pay attention to people, things, and events around them.

And being calm is harder for some babies than others, for two reasons.

The first reason is **neurobehavioural maturation**. Babies' nervous systems mature rapidly, but some babies are born less neurologically ready than others. Their nervous systems initially have a harder time adjusting to quick changes in sensory input, such as light, temperature, or sound. This makes them appear more "touchy" or "reactive."[21, 22]

The second reason is **temperament**, a set of tendencies each baby is born with that influence how he approaches, responds to, and interacts with the world.[20, 23, 24] Temperament is described along several scales like intensity, adaptability, rhythmicity, and activity. Temperament stays fairly stable over time, but can be shaped by life experiences. For example, babies who are easily distressed in unfamiliar situations are more likely to grow into fearful toddlers, while relaxed babies are more likely to become bold and sociable later on. However, temperament is not set in stone. Very few children remain extremely fearful or extremely bold: most move along the scale as they grow and have different experiences within their families and out in the world.[25] Temperament is how a baby responds to the world; it's only one component of a baby's personality, or who he is.

Some babies—approximately one out of ten—show distress quickly and intensely and are irregular and hard to soothe;[26] other babies are calmer and more predictable. But all babies cry, espe-cially in the early weeks. Interestingly, **patterns of crying** during the first year are remarkably similar across cultures, including the African !Kung, who always carry their babies and feed them completely on demand.[27] Babies in all cultures cry more during the first three months. The amount of crying remains about the same in the first six weeks and gradually decreases by twelve weeks. That being said, crying varies greatly from one baby to another: for example, in the first six weeks an average baby cries about two hours per day, but some babies cry as little as ten min-utes and others as much as four hours or more.[27, 28]

Healthy babies who cry more than three hours a day, more than three days a week, for over three weeks are considered colicky.[29] Colic usually starts a few days after birth (or after the expected due date for premature babies) and disappears by three months. Approximately one in four babies are described as col-icky at six weeks, and approximately one in ten at nine weeks.[27]

Colic is at the far end of the spectrum of crying, but it is still normal:[27]

- Colicky babies are very similar to non-colicky babies in feeding, weight gain, and family history of allergies.[29]
- Colicky babies tend to cry twice as much and more intensely during physical exams, but when scientists measured their physiological stress—heart rate and stress hormones—the levels were the same as those of non-colicky babies. In other words, colicky babies likely experience the same level of stress as non-colicky babies, but they express it more strongly.[30]
- There is no evidence that colic is an early sign of a more intense temperament.[30]

- Colicky babies are just as likely as non-colicky babies to have strong bonds with their parents.[31]

When babies are going through colic, they need extra support. Although it is currently unknown what exactly contributes to colic, there is some evidence of it being linked to overstimulation and insufficient sleep. Long crying spells tend to happen in the evenings when babies are more likely to be overstimulated and tired. Colicky babies sleep two hours a day less than average, and their internal rhythms are less coordinated.[30] Recently, researchers have used new molecular technologies and linked colic with microbiome imbalances: non-optimal composition of microorganisms in a baby's digestive system.[32, 33] A number of clinical trials tested the effectiveness of probiotics for reducing colic. Some probiotics were not effective, while others showed promise and need further research to confirm their benefits.[33, 34]

No amount of crying is easy for parents. Across cultures, hearing a baby cry activates specific areas in parents' brains in as fast as a hundred milliseconds: areas responsible for empathy, the urge to move, and the intention to speak.[35] Our drive to pick up and comfort a crying baby is universal, and that is a good thing.

Ready to connect

Newborns come into the world ready to connect and form relationships. According to attachment theory,[36, 37] each baby needs at least one person to whom she is strongly and mutually emotionally attached.[i]

A major misunderstanding surrounds this important concept. Many books and online resources take attachment to literally mean *physical* attachment. They tend to view "attachment parenting" as a set of specific practices and techniques such as babywearing, bed-sharing, and breastfeeding. Some or all of these practices may fit beautifully with your family, but they do not necessarily equal attachment. Attachment is *the quality of the relationship*. An attachment figure—a parent or a caregiver—helps baby regulate emotions and provides a sense of safety: a secure base from which baby explores the world.

Attachment = relationship quality (and not just techniques)

Research shows that secure attachment forms best when parents are *sensitive* and *mind-minded*. We will explore these concepts in more detail in Chapter 4, but I want to briefly touch on both here, because you will see them mentioned throughout the book.

Sensitivity is probably not a new concept for you. Sensitive parents and caregivers perceive, interpret, and respond to baby's signals in an accurate, prompt, and warm manner.

There is a good chance you have never heard of mind-mindedness, but it is something that matters, and something you can think about and even practice before your baby arrives. It comes from within the parent and can be learned.[38] Mind-minded parents and caregivers view their babies not just as little bundles of joy and potential, but as people with minds of their own.[39] Mind-minded parents tend to be more insightful, noticing and considering baby's emotions, sensations, and needs. They adjust their views and practices as they watch their baby's behaviour, rather than relying on pre-conceived notions, their own feelings and wishes, or general ideas of what babies need or should be doing.[40] In turn, babies whose parents are mind-minded tend to have a stronger physiological capacity to regulate their emotions[41]: it is easier for them to stay calm or return to a calm state. Later on, babies who grow in mind-minded environments tend to develop stronger bonds with their parents, learn to speak earlier, and recognize and understand emotions and needs of others around them more easily.[42, 43]

Ready to learn

Learning happens incredibly fast during the early months. At the core of learning is the ability to notice things that are interesting or new. And to be able to notice new things, very young babies need:

✓ More sleep
✓ Less stimulation when they're awake and alert

Does this seem counterintuitive? It will hopefully make sense to you in a moment. Fully noticing something involves more than simply seeing it with our eyes. To fully notice, or observe, something—an object, person, or an experience—a baby has to detect it, separate it from everything else, make some sense of it, and store it in memory.[9]

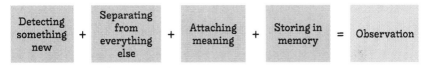

Good **sleep** is crucial for the first and last steps: a well-rested baby is calm and regulated when he's awake, which helps him detect new things around him; when he goes to sleep later on, his experiences are integrated into his memory.[44-46] And for the two steps in the middle, **less stimulation** is better than more. Excessive stimulation overwhelms baby's senses and quickly turns everything into a blur:[9]

• Bright lights block baby's ability to distinguish patterns, shapes, and colours

- Background noise louder than fifty decibels reduces baby's ability to hear differences in pitch, intensity, and sound patterns
- Strong odours like smoke and perfume overwhelm baby's nose and taste buds
- Baby's senses of touch, position, and movement develop early, but are easily overwhelmed by excessive stimulation (for example, a strongly vibrating baby seat)

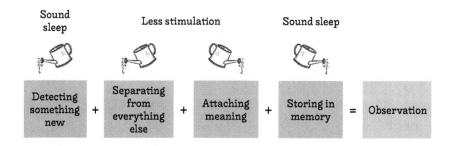

For babies who live in chaotic environments with a lot of noise, crowding, and unpredictability, noticing details is more difficult. For example, they tend to process complex visual stimuli more slowly. Researchers believe these babies may be chronically over-stimulated: they are living in a state of alertness and vigilance, but with reduced ability to pay attention to detail.[47]

Is there such thing as too little stimulation? In the first few weeks, the day-to-day care routines—feeding, diapering, bathing—are enough to fully engage a baby's senses and provide perfect opportunities for learning and connection. Because a baby is able to perceive and do more and more each day, she will continue to notice new elements in her environment as she grows.

We will explore how babies learn in more detail in Chapter 4, but in a nutshell, babies' brains constantly look for patterns in the world around them. They are making mental maps: "When I see this happen, I can expect that." They also look for surprise events that don't fit into the patterns they learned previously.[48] For example, by about five months babies learn that objects that are dropped usually fall down[49] and may be surprised to see a balloon floating in the air. Babies learn about the physical and social world around them by figuring out patterns and noticing new events. And it all begins in their home and family.

NEWBORNS: KEY POINTS

- Newborn babies are both competent and vulnerable.
- Every baby needs at least one person with whom they have a strong and mutual emotional attachment. Attachment forms best when parents and caregivers are sensitive and mind-minded.
- Young babies need *more* sleep and *less* stimulation for optimal learning.

PART II
GETTING READY FOR YOUR BABY

Getting ready for a new baby can be a very special and exciting time. Here I will describe what I believe are the most important things to prepare and think about: the minimum essential set. Once you have that in place, you can enjoy adding all the nice-to-haves, like cute clothes, a diaper bag, a stroller, baby carriers, and nursery decor.

Preparing your home

During pregnancy many families focus on staying healthy and preparing for the actual birth, but don't put enough thought into the postpartum period. However, the first few weeks after birth are very important for you and for your baby. I recommend that you decide on your baby's primary health care practitioner before your baby arrives. I also recommend that you gather your support system. Think about who you would like to see during the early postpartum days and weeks. Map out trusted local resources you might need or want, such as a postpartum doula and a lactation consultant.

When it comes to preparing your home, creating safe places for baby to sleep and feed at night is the most important step. Decide where your baby will sleep and how you will keep night feedings safe, and prepare these spaces in advance. Winging it or changing sleep approaches quickly out of one night's desperation because "nothing else works" can create unsafe environments for babies. You will find detailed advice on this in Chapter 2.

If you plan on driving with your baby, purchase and install a rear-facing infant car seat ahead of time. Learn how to adjust it and how to use it properly, and consult a car seat technician if you have questions.

Must-Haves Before Baby Arrives

Decide on:

- ✓ Baby's primary health care practitioner
- ✓ Your support system
- ✓ Where your baby will sleep (see pages 37–40 and 52–54)

Prepare:

- ✓ Safe place for sleep (see pages 52–58)
- ✓ Safe place for night feedings
- ✓ Formula and bottles if you will be formula-feeding
- ✓ Rear-facing infant car seat, properly installed if you have a vehicle
- ✓ 8 to 12 easy-on, breathable outfits
- ✓ Diapers and wipes
- ✓ 8 to 10 large receiving blankets

You will probably get many cute clothes for your baby. Make sure you have at least a few one-piece sleepers or gowns made of breathable materials like cotton, lyocell, modal, or bamboo. Those with zippers or snaps all the way down the front work best: you won't have to pull them over baby's head, which makes dressing much easier. It's also useful to have a stack of large flannel or muslin receiving blankets to double as burp cloths, stroller or baby-carrier shades, or nursing covers.

You might have heard that baby's nursery must have a black-and-white or a bright primary colour palette because babies can see contrasting colours best. But that's not really necessary. It's true that baby's vision is not fully developed at birth, but it improves rapidly: by two months she can scan her surroundings thoroughly and by six months she will see as well as an adult.[12, 50] Besides, in the early weeks, your baby doesn't yet need to see the details of the nursery. Seeing and feeling you is perfectly enough.

In fact, screening out more of the world's noise, brightness, and intensity will help your baby stay calmer and begin to focus her attention. Think about how your baby will experience your home. Are there adjustments you could make to turn the "volume" of everything down, to slow the pace? Consider decluttering, adding window drapes to soften light and sound, and moving away from background television (more on that in Chapter 4).

Bringing a new baby home, whether through pregnancy and birth or through adoption, is an enormous, life-changing event. Your mind and body will need time to adjust and recover. In some cultures there is a wonderful practice of a postpartum "babymoon" or "bubble" where mothers and babies stay home for twenty to forty days (often a moon cycle) after birth. Relatives help with chores, cooking, and hosting guests while the mother is given the space and time for deep rest and bonding with her newborn. This time is about nurturing mother and baby in their home and in their community.

The best gift I received after the birth of my second baby was from our circle of friends who brought delicious meals to us every few days for six weeks. It was absolutely amazing.

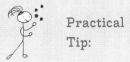

Practical
Tip:

How can you create a postpartum sanctuary, a protected space, if you live far away from family, have older children to care for, or must return to work? Try to gather your support system, do some planning, and create your own version of a postpartum bubble, if only for a short while. Only you can decide what it will look like and how long your "while" is. Arrange your life in a way that allows for as much rest and bonding with your baby as possible. Friends and family might offer to help with grocery shopping or caring for older children or pets. Ask for what you need most. Accept help—but only help that truly helps you. Step out of the superhuman expectations and try to keep your bubble intact. The early weeks are physically and emotionally demanding, but also special and precious like no other.

When you're out and about, family, friends, neighbours, and even strangers may ask to hold your baby. Don't feel like you have to say yes, especially during the cold and flu season. You might have heard that being held by others makes babies more social, or that exposure to germs strengthens baby's immune system. Neither of these is true. Your newborn doesn't yet benefit from social interactions: being held by the closest family is enough. Baby's immune system is not fully developed either, and his repertoire of immune responses is much smaller than that of an older child or adult.[51] Because of that, a virus that is "just a sniffle" to an adult can send a young baby to the hospital. What *does* strengthen baby's immune system is time and breastfeeding (more on that on pages 104–105). Your friends and family should understand if you err on the side of over-protectiveness for your newborn.

Preparing your mind

There may be no way to fully prepare your mind for the enormous change of becoming a parent and welcoming a new person into the world. But there are several key things to think about that will help you and your baby in the early weeks—and continue to matter for years to come.

The gift of being seen

Some of the best gifts you can give your baby are your intentional approach and your attention. Because babies can't talk yet, it's extra important we remain attentive, sensitive, and observant as we get to know them and learn to understand what they're communicating to us.

Tuning in is deliberate and not always easy. It is possible to love a baby and not be tuned into her needs or truly see her. It is also possible to be physically close to a baby and breeze through all the daily care activities, but not be tuned in. Sometimes we are so caught up in our thoughts or to-do lists that we forget to notice.

It might be hard for you to imagine what tuning in looks like if your baby has not yet arrived. Mind-mindedness, described earlier in this chapter, can help. Being mind-minded means *seeing baby as a whole person* and *considering baby's perspective*. It does not mean always knowing what baby needs—that would be impossible—but it does mean doing your best to put yourself in baby's shoes.

Next time you are around a baby or a young child, ask yourself how they might be feeling or what they might be thinking. Interestingly, this is often easier to do when you don't know the child; when you do know them, their temperament, likes, dislikes, or physical features tend to come to mind first: "She's always so active"; "He's such a good eater"; "What a cute baby." To practise mind-mindedness, try to focus on what the child might be feeling or thinking *in that moment* instead: "She might be overtired"; "I think he's really enjoying this apple sauce"; "This baby seems fascinated by the balloons."

Once your baby is here, you can practice mind-mindedness during your daily care routines. Your baby will be dependent on you, but not completely helpless. Think about how you could do things *with* your baby rather than *to* him. In the early days, get into the practice of telling your baby what you are about to do: "Let's change your diaper. I'm going to carry you to the changing table." Being talked to can be calming for a baby. In a study I briefly mentioned earlier, newborns' stress hormone levels dropped when they were massaged by a caregiver who made eye contact, spoke soothingly, and rocked them gently afterward. But when they were massaged in silence and without eye contact, they experienced a stress hormone surge, just like babies undergoing painful procedures.[16] So, speaking to your baby when you take care of him can make a difference in how your baby feels. It also sets the stage for future interactions. For example, your older baby will begin participating in diaper changes by cooing, holding a clean diaper, and lifting his bottom. I deliberately chose to not have toys in the changing area or hang a mobile over it, so that my babies and me could interact more easily and experience the care routines together.

Another way to practice mind-mindedness is to simply be with your baby. Hold your baby or lie down next to her and watch her quietly. Try not to think about what you want her to do or what the charts say she's supposed to be doing at this age; see her in the moment, as she is. Notice what she's looking at, what she's working on, and what might be hard for her.

As you observe your baby, you will notice these states:[52]

- Quiet alert: baby is not moving much and is focusing intently on people and objects around her; this is a period of intense learning and interaction; you might notice your baby turning toward the sound of your voice or trying to mimic your facial expressions.
- Active alert: baby is moving actively.
- Drowsy: baby is transitioning between awake and asleep (yawning, droopy eyelids).
- Deep sleep: baby is sleeping quietly and is fully relaxed.
- Light sleep: baby's eyelids are fluttering and she's moving around in her sleep.
- Crying.

Of these states, crying, of course, is the easiest to recognize. When your baby cries, he is telling you about his state and asking for engagement. In a sense, crying is your baby's first language: this is how he communicates hunger, thirst, pain, discomfort, fatigue, and overstimulation. A baby communicating his needs by crying is not necessarily in distress. Most of the time he is asking for a change in his environment: a feeding, a clean diaper, less stimulation, or an opportunity to sleep. Crying is a clue to his needs. Answering a baby's cry absolutely never "spoils" him; it teaches him that he is safe and that his needs will be met.

Babies who cry often and are hard to soothe are sometimes called "difficult," whereas calmer babies are described as "easy." I believe it is better to stay away from generalized labels like these, because they're subjective and may bring feelings of guilt or unmet expectations. Instead, try to think of a baby being *unsettled* (as opposed to *content*) *in this moment*. This mindset will help you focus on what your baby might be telling you and how you could adjust her environment to better meet her needs.

That being said, it can be helpful to think about your baby's overall temperament as she grows, so you can understand her better and predict and plan for circumstances that might be hard for her. For example, a child who is more intense and less adaptable may need extra time to prepare for a new experience or a change in routine.

The power of routines

Many of us consider ourselves spontaneous, but if you think about it, we all have quite a few routines: activities that occur in the same order and about the same time each day.[53] Some routines are obvious and others are more subtle. Do you generally follow the same steps when making breakfast or getting ready for work? What about getting ready for bed? Routines simplify our days, keep us grounded, and bring a sense of well-being and comfort. And routines may be even more important to babies.

 From Your Baby's Perspective:

Imagine you are riding a train in an unfamiliar area; all you know is the name of your destination. You probably keep watching the announcements, trying to gauge how soon you should get ready to disembark, perhaps feeling alert and a bit tense.

For our babies, every day feels like that unfamiliar train ride: things are changing rapidly around them and they have little control over it. Even their bodies are constantly changing as they grow and master new skills! Changes, transitions, and novelty can be overwhelming, but routines can help. Babies' brains are looking for patterns and they soon begin recognizing the steps of the routine. This helps babies predict what comes next and feel safe and calm.

I think of routines as sequences of events that are woven into the day to make it more predictable and cozy. For example, a baby can learn and anticipate the familiar steps of a bedtime routine: after a warm bath he will get a fresh diaper and pyjamas, help draw the shades, hear a lullaby, feed, and be gently placed down to sleep. Being able to predict what comes next helps baby stay calmer and develop an inner rhythm more easily.

Another benefit of routines is that they provide early opportunities for babies to take part in a shared activity. Moving through routines together in a multisensory way—with baby holding the wash cloth, lifting arms to put pyjamas on, or waving goodnight—and repeating the steps daily helps create a rich environment for early learning.[54]

Does this mean you should put your baby on a schedule as early as possible? Definitely not. On-the-clock, rigid schedules are a construct of the adult world. Asking or forcing babies to conform to adult schedules would not be sensitive to their needs. Instead, you can help your baby establish an inner rhythm by carefully watching her cues and structuring the day around her needs: feeding her when she is hungry, making sure conditions are conducive for napping at the time she needs to sleep, and gradually developing routines around these events. Over time, your baby will settle into a more predictable rhythm that *you* can now anticipate. In a sense, you will develop routines and rhythms together with your baby.

In the next chapter we will talk about developing rhythms and routines around what can be one of the biggest challenges of the early parenting months or even years: sleep.

CHAPTER 2
SLEEP

"How old is she?"

"Eighteen weeks," I answered proudly; a new mom, still counting in weeks.

"Is she a good baby?"

"She is wonderful... amazing."

"You're so lucky! Neither of mine slept well when they were this little."

Oh. I hadn't realized that's what the question was about... I was much too tired.

C hances are, someone has already asked or will soon ask you this question: is your baby "good"? So I will say this right at the start: your baby's sleep is *not* indicative of his future or personality, or his "goodness," even if there were such a thing. Neither is it a measure of you as a parent, if there were such a measure. Sleep is simply a biological need, yours and your baby's. Your family will find your path to it; this chapter is meant to make that path shorter.

If you're asking yourself, "What is healthy sleep?," "What should I expect at this stage?," or "When will my baby sleep through the night?," you are not alone. In a survey completed in the 1990s, almost half of all parents expressed the need for more information on children's sleep.[55] Is this still true today, with so much information at our fingertips? Yes, and perhaps even more so. The most common questions pediatricians receive from parents are about sleep challenges, and yet most health care professionals have minimal training in children's sleep.[56-58] When we turn to books, online articles, or social networks, we find a lot of advice. It varies in philosophy, principles, and beliefs about the needs of babies and the "right" baby care, and is often contradictory and confusing.[59]

Two sleep approaches that stem from seemingly opposite ideas are "intuitive parenting" and "infant behaviour management."[60] You may have heard about these under the names of attachment parenting (or "wait it out") and sleep training (or "cry it out"). The attachment parenting approach suggests soothing baby to sleep and responding to night wakings for as long as needed. The sleep-training approach recommends teaching baby to fall asleep unassisted and encouraging self-soothing. Hundreds of resources strongly advocate for one approach and harshly criticize the other. I promised you to not bring parenting wars into this book and I will keep that promise. If you haven't yet read the conflicting sleep advice, try to avoid it. If you have, try to set it aside. I trust that all parents, no matter what sleep philosophy they choose, want to meet their baby's needs *and* strengthen their bond with their baby. I believe we can do both, and do so without any particular sleep philosophy other than that of love, respect, intention, and knowledge. We can do it by understanding sleep, being intentional and thoughtful in creating the sleep environments in our homes, and carefully watching our own, unique babies.

But why would we need to create a sleep environment at all? Don't babies learn to sleep naturally, just like they learn to walk?

The truth is, babies do have the ability to sleep well early on,[61] but the setup, the pace, and the ever-changing patterns of our modern lives often interfere with the unfolding of this natural, biological process. What we do, and how we do it, can disrupt sleep and mask baby's natural sleep abilities.

 From Your Baby's
Perspective:

Imagine you are learning to drive a car. You see that most people around you drive well, seemingly naturally, so you figure it can't be too hard. However, every time you practice, you're in a different vehicle and the road rules have changed. Some days the instructor is there and does most of the driving for you, but other days he leaves you on your own. You also have to practise late in the day when you're tired. I suspect you'd still learn to drive despite these challenges, but it might not happen as fast or as easily as you had hoped.

This is what it might be like for a baby who is figuring out how to get the rest he needs in a busy environment. He sleeps in different places under different conditions; sometimes his parents are over-helping—for example, by rocking or bouncing him to sleep— and sometimes under-helping,[62] suddenly leaving him to fall asleep on his own.

Adults are accustomed to the fast pace, lack of rhythm, and high demands of our society, and this is reflected in mainstream baby sleep advice. Many parenting books recommend doing whatever it takes to help baby fall asleep in the first four months and then considering sleep training, such as letting baby "cry it out." But there is another way. I will help you create the environment that supports sleep, and guide you in helping your baby *begin sleeping well as early as he can*—without crying it out, but with some upfront effort and commitment from you. I will also explain why many commonly believed "facts" about baby sleep are actually baby sleep myths.

Baby Sleep Myths

Myth #1: *Putting baby to bed later will help baby sleep in.*

Myth #2: *Cutting out naps will make baby sleep better at night.*

Myth #3: *Babies can easily sleep on the go, especially if we tire them out.*

Myth #4: *Switching to formula and introducing solid foods will help baby sleep better.*

Myth #5: *There is no point in being consistent; teething will throw everything off anyway.*

Tempting as it may be to skip straight to Part II of this chapter, especially if your baby is already here, I encourage you to read Part I first to understand—truly understand—your baby's sleep. This understanding will give you a solid foundation for creating your baby's sleep environment and practices, now and as your baby grows.

First, let's take a look at the science behind sleep patterns: what they are, how they develop, and what helps and hinders babies' sleep.

PART I
UNDERSTANDING SLEEP

C onsider this: your baby will spend more than half of her first year of life asleep.[63] By the time she's three years old, she will still likely have spent more time sleeping than in all her wakeful activities combined.[64] Why do young children sleep so much?

The role of sleep

We all know that sleep brings physical rest and restoration. A lesser known fact is that sleep also involves intense brain activity,[44,65] especially in babies. During certain phases of sleep your baby's brain works hard, re-playing and processing experiences of the day and integrating them into memory[44-46]—remember the "How babies learn" diagram on page 10? As Dr. Avi Sadeh says in his book *Sleeping Like a Baby*,[61] a baby's brain is like a librarian who spends the day busily helping visitors and only gets a chance to carefully examine, sort, and organize the materials in his care after the library closes. Neuroscientists believe that the different phases of sleep uniquely contribute to learning and emotional regulation.[66-68]

Does the quality of sleep affect development? If we set very rare cases of extreme sleep deprivation aside and look at most babies' sleep and development, the answer is... yes and no. Overall, scientific literature suggests that there is an *association* between sleep and mental and physical development:[69] babies who sleep better are usually a bit further ahead. Positive associations have also been found beyond babyhood: better sleep at twelve months has been found to be associated with better attention regulation and fewer behavioural problems later on when babies grew into preschoolers.[70] However, there's not enough data to prove sleep *caused* these differences.[63] In other words, well-rested babies are generally further ahead in their development, but we cannot confidently conclude that sleep, or sleep alone, is the reason for that.

What about the effects of sleep on growth? Back in the 1960s scientists discovered that growth hormones in young children are produced mainly during sleep, especially during deep sleep in the evening hours.[71] This tells us that sleep and physical growth are indeed linked physiologically. One study found that six-month-old babies who slept well were taller than babies who didn't sleep well.[72] However, once again, no studies so far have proven that poor sleep *causes* growth problems.

Several studies point to the link between sleep quality and metabolic and immune system functioning in adults.[73,74] It is reasonable to expect this to be true for young children and babies as well.

Finally, what about behaviour and emotions? Most of us have experienced the effects of poor sleep on our own ability to focus and to stay unruffled during challenging situations. A recent study found that the more attentive and sensitive mothers were toward their babies, the more advanced their babies' behavioural, emotional, and cognitive development was later on—but this was true only for babies who got enough sleep![75,76] In other words, babies can be too tired to fully benefit from positive experiences. (As the authors of one of the studies aptly titled their paper, "My

mother is sensitive, but I am too tired to know"[76].) 28
think, is important.

To me, the best way to summarize the role of sl
sound sleep helps babies' natural development unfold
healthy nutrition, gives them a strong base upon which to grow.

Next, let's take a look at the *nature* of sleep: the things about
our babies' sleep we cannot change, but can benefit from knowing about.

How sleep works

Sleep structure—the way all humans sleep—is regulated by the
internal body rhythms created by homeostatic, circadian, and
ultradian drives. Homeostatic drive, also called sleep pressure,
makes us progressively sleepier the longer we stay awake and less
able to stay asleep the longer we sleep. If it were the only process regulating our sleep, we would have a really hard time staying awake in the evening and have trouble sleeping in the early
morning hours. What helps us here is the circadian drive, also
known as our biological clock. Regulated by the hormone melatonin, it works in opposition to the homeostatic drive and makes
us more wakeful as the day progresses and sleepier as the night
goes on. The balance between these two drives allows adults to
function on a twenty-four-hour basis by having about eight hours
of consolidated sleep at night and staying awake for about sixteen
hours during the day.[77] Finally, we have the ultradian drive which
creates the rhythm between the phases of sleep. During non-rap-
id-eye-movement (non-REM) sleep, our bodies and minds rest
quietly and restore. In REM sleep, our physiological systems are
more active; this is when we experience most of our dreams. As
the night goes on we cycle back and forth between periods of

non-REM and REM sleep. A sleep cycle of an adult lasts about ninety to a hundred minutes.

But in the first four to six months, babies sleep quite differently from older children and adults.[28] What happens in those early months?

Week 1: Baby received high levels of melatonin from his mother before birth. This melatonin keeps him extra sleepy most of the day and night.

Weeks 2–12: After the first week, the borrowed melatonin has dissipated and "day-night confusion" often sets in: baby begins sleeping in short stretches around the clock or sleeps more during the day than at night. His circadian rhythm has not yet developed, so he goes to sleep when he's tired and wakes up as soon as his drive to sleep diminishes, taking naps at all hours. Between six and twelve weeks baby begins to make melatonin himself, but the levels are still low.[29] His developing sleep rhythms may not be in sync with each other: waking and sleeping states may overlap, be incomplete, or switch rapidly. Wakeful but tired, baby may cry a lot. Some researchers believe that immature sleep rhythms and the resulting tiredness are one of the major reasons for the inconsolable crying we know as colic.[30]

At this age, when your baby goes to sleep, she spends the first ten minutes or so in lighter REM sleep and then enters a stretch of deep sleep. This is why a baby who falls asleep in your arms may wake up if you attempt to shift position or put her down right away.

At the same time, baby is quickly developing an ability to sleep long stretches known in the scientific literature as *the longest sustained sleep period*. This developing ability to sleep longer stretches—the consolidation of sleep—is intrinsic: it is biologically determined in all human babies. The numbers are very consistent across different studies: the longest sleep period, on average, is 3.6 hours at three weeks, 5.2 hours at eight weeks, and 6 hours at twelve weeks.[80-82] As the sleep periods lengthen, the number of night wakings predictably goes down, from an average of four wakings per night at four weeks to two to three wakings at nine weeks.[83]

Weeks 12–16 (3–4 months): Baby's melatonin levels are now high enough for a clear circadian rhythm to be established,[79, 84, 85] ending the day-night confusion. The longest sleep period shifts to nighttime and can be as long as six hours.[80, 82] When baby goes to sleep, she now enters a stretch of deeper non-REM sleep right away and overall spends much more time in deep, quiet sleep than she did in the early weeks.[86] Her sleep cycle is now about forty minutes long. If you had a polysomnograph and could watch your sleeping baby's brain waves as scientists do in the lab, you would now see patterns called sleep spindles and K-complexes. Your baby has completed the transition from neonatal to infant sleep.[86] Such an amazing amount of change in a short period of time, isn't it?

After 16 weeks (4 months): At this point, there are no more biologically determined big changes in baby's sleep! Baby's longest sleep period stops lengthening on its own and remains at four to seven hours.[80, 82] Similarly, the typical number of night wakings stays at two to three per night.[83, 87] The homeostatic and ultradian drives do continue to mature slowly through toddlerhood and beyond. Homeostatic sleep pressure will begin to build and dissipate more slowly, leading to a lesser need for daytime naps; because of this, babies stop napping at some point between three and six years old. As the ultradian drive matures, the length of a baby's sleep cycle will gradually increase from forty minutes to ninety to a hundred minutes by school age.[88] But overall, once a baby develops distinct sleep cycles and consolidates most of her sleep into nighttime—usually by four months and almost always by six months—*her sleep biology will remain fairly constant throughout her life.*[88, 89]

Take a look at the chart on the next page. It shows a sleep pattern of a child I will call Eva. On this typical night, Eva fell asleep just after 7 p.m. and slept deeply until around 10 p.m. She woke up around 10:30 p.m., tossed and turned at around 1 a.m., woke again at 2 a.m., and tossed and turned at 3 a.m. and 5 a.m. She then had another period of deep sleep and got up for the day around 7 a.m.

Armed with your new knowledge of baby sleep development, can you guess how old Eva is? Yes, she could be six months old— or six years old. Her biological sleep pattern has been in place since she was a four-month-old baby.

Looking at the chart, you might wonder:

1. Eva woke up twice, yet, she could be six years old. Why is she still not sleeping through the night?
2. Eva had two periods of deep sleep—in the evening and during the early morning hours—with a stretch of light sleep in between. Her light sleep and her wakings, ironically, overlapped almost exactly with the time her parents were probably sleeping themselves. Wouldn't parents get more sleep if Eva went to bed later, so that her first period of deep sleep overlapped with her parents' sleep more?

Let's look at both questions more closely—they are important.

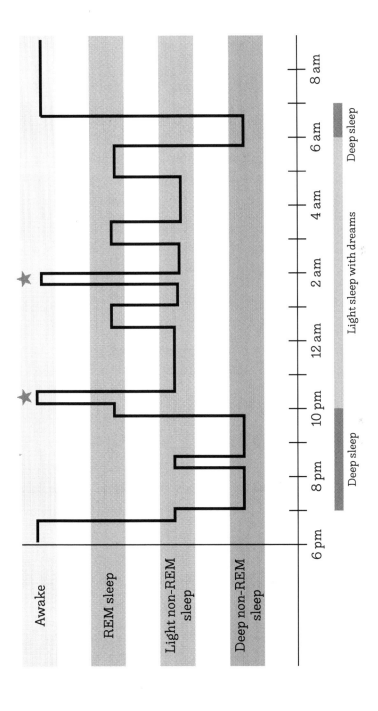

Typical night sleep of a child. Common wakings are marked with stars; the child might also wake up during each period of REM sleep. (Adapted from Adair and Bauchner [1993][90] and Ferber [2006][89].)

Sleeping through the night

In our Western culture, we consider a good sleeper to be a baby who sleeps through the night. But what does sleeping through the night really mean? According to the most accepted scientific definition, it means sleeping between 12 a.m. and 5 a.m. for six or more nights per week, over four consecutive weeks.[91] So, if you come across a statement that says most babies sleep through the night by four months (and yours doesn't), remember that they're talking about a five-hour stretch: certainly not what most adults consider a full night of sleep.

But is there such thing as sleeping through the night in the first place? Not in the "sleeping continuously in one, long stretch" sense. All of us, babies and adults alike, tend to wake briefly after a stretch of REM sleep and become more aware of our environment. If all seems well, we turn over, peacefully return to sleep, and most likely don't recall this brief waking when we get up for the day. Interestingly, this was not known until the late 1970s. By videotaping babies, Dr. Thomas Anders and his research team were the first to discover that all babies wake up at night, even those who, according to their parents, "sleep through."[81, 92]

Remember the biologically determined *longest sustained sleep period*, which lengthens on its own by four months because of sleep consolidation and then stays at around four to seven hours? We can now start talking about *the longest self-regulated sleep period*—a period of quietude that includes both sleep and calm wakefulness during brief wakings.[82] Essentially, this is the length of time your baby is in bed, sleeping or resting quietly. Once your baby develops the ability to sustain sleep for longer stretches, go back to sleep calmly after brief wakings, and consistently do so during what your family considers nighttime,[82] your baby is "sleeping through the night." When a baby takes night feedings, but goes back to sleep quickly and easily, some consider this "sleeping through" and others do not. I like to think of it as *sound sleep*.

You see, night wakings themselves are not a problem and are completely natural. Most restless nights are due to difficulties *getting back to sleep* after waking, not the waking itself. Night wakings are also not something baby will simply grow out of. Sleeping through the night requires not only intrinsic, biological sleep maturation, but also sleep regulation—baby's ability to initiate and re-initiate sleep on their own[93]—something you've probably heard about as "**self-soothing**."

Baby's natural ability to sleep for long stretches develops quickly over the first few months, but does not improve much afterward. Sleeping for longer than four to seven hours becomes possible because baby is now able to go back to sleep on her own, not because of a change in her sleep structure.

The term "self-soothing" was introduced by the same researchers who first discovered that all babies wake up at night. They called babies who cried "signallers," and babies who went back to sleep on their own "self-soothers."[94, 95] This observation, or the term itself, didn't imply that babies need to be left to cry to become self-soothers. However, since then much controversy has grown around it. Do babies need to *learn* to self-soothe? Is "crying it out" the only way to learn? Is it harmful to babies? We will get back to these questions in Part II of this chapter. For now, consider this: the longest self-regulated sleep period has been found to always be longer than the longest sustained sleep period, even in very young babies.[82] This means that most babies are capable of re-settling to sleep on their own when they are as young as a month old. In fact, in one study, one-month-olds re-initiated sleep on their own in one out of every three wakings.[83] This tells us that babies already have the ability to initiate sleep on their own at one month of age, and possibly even from birth.

You probably want to see some hopeful sleep numbers. Taken together, night sleep and naps add up to thirteen to sixteen hours per day for most babies.[96] Studies of babies sleeping on their own show that 53 percent of them sleep eight-hour stretches at night by six months, and 72 percent by twelve months. Many babies can self-regulate sleep for over ten hours by twelve months.[82]

Early to bed, early to rise

But let's go back to Eva's sleep example. Just like other babies and young children, Eva has her longest stretch of sleep in the evening. Shouldn't her parents put her to bed later, when they go to bed themselves, so that their deep sleep overlaps?

The thing is, baby's biological clock is pre-set for getting up early even when she goes to bed late. One study looked at sleep of almost thirty thousand children from birth to age three living in seventeen different countries. Although their typical bedtimes varied greatly—from 7:30 p.m. in New Zealand to 10:20 p.m. in Hong Kong—children in all countries woke early, generally between 6 and 8 a.m. Bedtime was the best predictor of total night sleep duration.[97] In other words, a baby who goes to sleep late will likely get fewer hours of night sleep and miss some of the deep sleep that typically happens in the evening hours.

What about the babies who wake up *really early*, at 4 or 5 a.m.? For most babies, this is a natural waking point at the end of a REM sleep period (see Eva's brief waking at around 5 a.m.?). By that point, the baby has already had a good amount of rest and her homeostatic drive to sleep is not very strong, so she may wake fully and want to get up for the day. However, this waking could be followed by another hour or more of deep sleep,[90] just like in Eva's example. Getting up before 6 a.m. may rob baby of deep, restorative sleep.

A good sleeper

What makes a good sleeper? Contrary to some beliefs, baby boys and girls sleep equally well.[81, 98-100] Similarly, bigger babies and those described as "happy" don't seem to sleep significantly better than their smaller or more touchy peers.[83] But sleep does come easier to some babies than others. As Dr. William Sears points out in *The Baby Book*, "good sleepers are partly born, partly made, never forced" and science supports that. Babies are born with varying degrees of neurological maturity, or "readiness," which is not a predictor of future development or personality, but which does seem to predict sleep. Babies with higher neurological maturity at birth—measured as the percentage of time they spent in quiet sleep—were found to sleep better at twelve months.[83] But neurological maturity and other pre-set factors aren't the only things that influence sleep. Studies of twins show that genetics is responsible for up to 50 percent of differences in sleep patterns—and environment is responsible for the other 50 percent.[99, 101]

When a new baby joins your family, you don't know what kind of sleep predisposition he comes with—and even if you did, you couldn't do anything about it anyway. But no matter what kind of little sleeper you have, there's a lot you can do to support his sleep, helping him sleep as soundly as possible.

What affects sleep

Let's now take a look at the *nurture* of sleep: how the environment we create and our daily practices affect our babies' sleep. I have to begin by saying that most studies on the effects of the physical environment and care on babies' sleep have been done in Western countries, and the majority of these studies focused on babies who were sleeping on their own (not bed-sharing with a parent). In this section I cover sleep practices relevant to all families, whether they bed-share or their babies sleep solo, but with a focus on the home environment of a typical Western family.

In addition, sleep research mostly focuses on mothers and babies. The role of fathers in sleep-related care, and baby care in general, remains a relatively unexplored topic in science. Some researchers note that they focused on the mothers because only a few fathers in their studies were spending enough time with babies at bedtime to yield usable data.[102] I think most findings on the effects of baby care done by moms also apply to caring dads and other close caregivers: their roles just haven't been studied enough yet.

Sleeping position

If there is one topic that all researchers and practitioners agree on, it's this: babies should be placed to sleep on their backs. Babies have likely been put to sleep on a parent's chest or beside a parent on their side or back throughout much of human history for safety and breastfeeding. In the 1950s, Dr. Benjamin Spock and other practitioners began recommending putting babies to sleep on their tummies; this advice, based on untested theories, tragically coincided with a big rise in Sudden Infant Death Syndrome (SIDS) rates in Western countries through the 1970s and 1980s. In the 1990s, Back-to-Sleep campaigns began to urge parents to put babies to sleep on their backs again—and SIDS rates went down.[103] We now know that babies sleeping on their tummies spend more time in deep sleep[104] and have a harder time arousing from it, which puts them at a greater risk for SIDS.[105] Babies sleep more lightly on their backs, but they evolved to sleep lightly for a reason: they need to be able to wake up if they face any physiological difficulties. This is especially true for premature babies and babies younger than four months.[78]

Sleep arrangement

Babies around the world sleep in many different environments. Some babies sleep alone in their own rooms (I will call this *solo sleeping*). Other babies *co-sleep* with their parents, siblings, or other family members by sharing the same sleep environment. Of these co-sleeping babies, some also *bed-share* (sleep with an adult on the same surface), while others only *room-share* (sleep in the same room, but on a different surface, such as a crib or bassinet).[106] The terms co-sleeping and bed-sharing are often used interchangeably, but they mean different things. When you're looking at research or recommendations, be sure to take note of what's being referred to: *sharing the room* or *sharing the bed*.

A number of studies have looked at the benefits and risks associated with bed-sharing. Documented benefits include higher breastfeeding rates and better milk supply for mom, more stable heart rate and breathing patterns for baby, and more consistent responses to baby's cues.[107] Research on risks suggests that bed-sharing itself is not hazardous, but the circumstances in which it occurs can be.[108,109] Sharing the sleep surface has physiological benefits and has been a historical norm for many centuries. However, over the past couple hundred years our society has changed, and some of these changes have made bed-sharing unsafe. One study analyzed a large amount of data from SIDS studies and concluded that bed-sharing significantly increases the risk of SIDS; the results suggested that about 90% of bed-sharing SIDS deaths would likely not have occurred had the baby not been bed-sharing.[110] However, a study that followed[109] re-analyzed the same data and found that, in the absence of hazards such as sleeping with an adult on a sofa or chair, or with an adult who had consumed more than two units of alcohol, who had taken medication, or who smoked, bed-sharing did not significantly increase the SIDS rate. This important and well-designed study has received a lot of media attention and eased the minds of many parents who are bed-sharing or who plan to do it in the future. However, it is very important to understand that this study looked at SIDS cases only—in other words, cases when the cause of infant death could not be determined. Cases of accidental asphyxiation (from being laid on by a person or object or from becoming wedged in the structure of the bed) and cases of hyperthermia (overheating) were not included. The risks bed-sharing poses for these outcomes are, therefore, unknown.

A study that conclusively tells us once and for all whether bed-sharing is *absolutely* safe will never be possible because nothing can ever be proven completely safe (or *be* completely safe, for that matter). It is critically important that parents who plan on bed-sharing research the options thoroughly to make sure their sleeping arrangement is as safe as possible in their particular circumstances. Extra care must be taken in the first four months when SIDS risks are the greatest.

The majority of pediatric professionals recommend babies sleep on their own sleeping surface.[59] The current recommendation of the American Academy of Pediatrics (AAP) is to room-share, but not bed-share, with your baby during the first year.[111] In practice, this usually means baby is sleeping in a crib or a bassinet beside her parents' bed.

Benefits of safe bed-sharing:
easier breastfeeding, physiological benefits, bonding.
Benefits of baby sleeping solo:
safety, parents' sleep quality, grown-up time.

When it comes to baby's sleep quality, where baby sleeps does not seem to matter as long as it's safe. Bed-sharing has been linked to slightly more fragmented sleep in some studies,[112-114] but in other studies it did not affect babies' sleep quality or amount when practised consistently.[115-117] In one study, bed-sharing babies had more frequent but shorter awakenings during the night, so in total they slept for just as long as solo-sleeping babies.[115] Another study found that co-sleeping and solo-sleeping three- and six-month-olds did not differ in any sleep measures (total night-time sleep duration, longest sleep period, time awake during the night, or number of wakings lasting five minutes or more); co-sleeping moms did not get as much nighttime sleep as moms of solo-sleeping babies, but they napped more and did not feel less rested overall.[117] Parents who intentionally choose to co-sleep often explain their decision by mentioning the value of closeness, while those who choose solo sleeping for their babies often mention the value of independence.[118]

What about the link between sleep arrangements and sleep problems? There is evidence that families who intentionally and proactively make the decision to bed-share early on, due to cultural traditions or caregiving beliefs, are usually happy with the practice. However, families who do not plan to bed-share but who reactively switch to it, often report sleep problems and general dissatisfaction with their sleep arrangement.[119-121] In fact, many of these "reactive" families turned to bed-sharing as the last resort because of an existing sleep problem.[59] And contrary to a popular belief, bed-sharing during babyhood does not seem to be predictive of bed-sharing later in childhood.[114] Overall, these studies tell us that bed-sharing itself is not likely to cause sleep problems.

In recent years, even the polar opposite experts on baby sleep have moved closer to the middle, to the position that *where* a baby sleeps is not nearly as important as the *interactions* during the transitions to and from sleep.[59] We will look at these interactions next.

Practices that help sound sleep

In the early weeks, the most helpful sleep-related practices are those that support the development of baby's sleep structure. For example, natural outdoor light during the day and darkness at night help circadian rhythm development.[79,122] Babies who are not exposed to electronic screens tend to sleep better.[123,124] Breastfeeding, besides having other important benefits, also helps babies sleep: breastmilk contains sleep-inducing hormone melatonin at night,[125] with a peak between midnight and 4 a.m., and no detectable melatonin during the day.[126]

There is growing and consistent evidence that sleep development happens more rapidly and naturally in calm environments with low stimulation. Although much of this research focused on premature babies, it likely applies to full-term babies in the early months as well. Low-stimulating, rhythmic care was found to result in better defined sleep and alert states, more quiet sleep, and less fussing and crying.[127] An excessively stimulated young baby may fall asleep as a way to avoid overstimulation.[128] Come to think of it, it's his only way to escape! If this happens regularly, his natural sleep cycle development and sleep consolidation may become disrupted.

After the first few weeks, practices that support baby's ability to transition between sleep cycles also become important. As we saw earlier, sleeping through the night, or sleeping well in general, does not mean sleeping in one continuous stretch. Instead, sound sleep involves smoothly going back to sleep after brief wakings between sleep cycles. Remember that many babies have the ability to re-initiate sleep on their own, or re-settle, when they are only a month old?[82] In a study that followed babies through their first year, 57 percent gradually began sleeping better by re-settling on their own more, but 43 percent re-settled on their own *less* over time.[83] Why did some babies develop this ability further while others seemed to have forgotten it?

If we look to science, it can tell us quite a bit about what practices support re-settling. Two "ingredients" are very consistent across numerous studies:

✓ Consistent sleep associations and routines
✓ Balanced daily rhythm

Consistent sleep associations and routines

Sleep associations, or sleep cues, are people, things, and events that a baby associates with falling asleep and getting back to sleep. Babies who consistently experience the same sleep associations when they go to sleep at bedtime and when they wake up in the middle of the night are much more likely to re-settle on their own.[89, 129]

From Your Baby's
Perspective:

Imagine you go to sleep as usual, on your favourite side of the bed, with your usual blanket and pillow. You wake up at night to find that your pillow is no longer there. You sit up to check if it somehow fell on the floor... and realize you are not even in your bedroom, but rather in the living room. Imagine this happening several times in a row, and each time you find yourself in a different part of your home. You're probably not going to roll over and go back to sleep; you're likely to be wide awake, trying to figure out where you are.

This is how a baby might feel when she falls asleep in one place and wakes up in another.

Matching going-to-bed associations with middle-of-the-night ones can take many different forms. For example, a baby who bed-shares and falls asleep next to a parent will likely expect to find a parent next to her in the middle of the night. If she always goes to sleep nursing, she will likely want to nurse when she wakes up. A baby who falls asleep with a pacifier is likely to look for it in the middle of the night. For a baby sleeping in her own room, re-settling independently at night is easier if she consistently falls asleep on her own at bedtime. Many studies from around the world have shown that babies who go to sleep without an adult in the room are more likely to be able to re-settle without help during the night.[97, 130]

Babies re-settle on their own more when given brief opportunities and space to practise.[83, 131] When researchers videotape sleeping babies, they see that most make at least some attempts to re-settle on their own[95]: some by sucking their thumb or fingers, others by moving their heads side to side. After these attempts babies may or may not call out. When parents wait a few minutes before picking a baby up, he may re-settle on his own. And waiting may be a good idea for another reason. Babies can suck, smile, or even cry a bit during REM sleep, so they appear to be awake, but they are not.[121] Swooping in right away can wake a baby who was sleeping, interrupting his sleep cycle.

Babies sometimes suck, smile, or even cry a bit in their sleep. Swooping in right away may wake a baby who was sleeping.

Consistent bedtime and nap time routines—sequences of events that take place before baby goes to sleep—create calmer bedtimes. Because baby's brain seeks patterns and learns what to expect from the world through repetition,[48, 132] routines and rituals bring a sense of knowing what is happening next and are reassuring and calming.

Are some routines better than others? Research shows that *what* happens during bedtime routines—cuddling, quiet activities, feeding—does not seem to affect how well babies sleep.[102] But *how* bedtime routines are done does correlate with sleep. Babies whose mothers were emotionally available at bedtime—sensitive and responsive to their babies' cues—were found to sleep better, probably because their mothers helped them relax and trust their environment.[102]

Balanced daily rhythm

Day and night sleep are connected parts of the overall sleep structure and the flow of the day. Adjusting the daily rhythm by giving baby consistent, predictable opportunities for naps improves both day and night sleep.[133] Naps are opportunities for physical rest and memory consolidation (remember the librarian analogy?) built into each day.

You may wonder why baby needs consistent naps. If she did not have a chance to nap at her usual time, wouldn't she simply catch a longer nap later? Unfortunately, most babies who miss their nap window become too tired and have trouble falling asleep later. This "too tired" state is often called being "overtired."

From Your Baby's
Perspective:

Think of a time when you had to catch a red-eye flight or to study all night long. Even if you had a chance to get some sleep in the morning, you probably didn't fall asleep easily. That's because in response to fatigue your body turned up the production of chemicals that are responsible for keeping you alert, such as cortisol.[121] Your body assumed there must be a good reason for you to be awake.

This is what happens to a baby who misses a nap.

One day researchers might find that different degrees of sleep deficit—ranging from mild overtiredness and short-term lack of sleep to long-term sleep deprivation—produce different chemical imbalances. What we do know at this point is that well-rested babies sleep better. As Dr. Marc Weissbluth says in *Healthy Sleep Habits, Happy Child*, "sleep begets sleep."

When a baby is well-rested, the rhythms created by the homeostatic, circadian, and ultradian processes are in sync, making it easier for him to stay alert when awake and relaxed when asleep. It also helps baby transition between sleep cycles with only a brief waking, which in turn helps develop self-settling.

Can a baby compensate for lost night sleep by napping more? Research tells us that babies who wake up more at night or who go to bed late do tend to take more frequent or longer naps, but they don't fully catch up: their total sleep is still reduced.[97,120] Naps are also a bit different from night sleep. Naps contain less REM sleep than night sleep does,[80] with more REM sleep in a morning nap compared to an afternoon one.[65]

As babies grow, they are able to stay awake longer. On average, the longest awake span is approximately two hours for babies under three months old, 2.5 hours by 4.5 months, and 3.5 hours by six months.[80] However, remember that these are the *longest* awake spans, which usually happen between the last nap of the day and bedtime.[80] Many sleep resources recommend a two-hour awake window for young babies, so many parents *begin* soothing their babies for a nap after two hours (I made this mistake myself). But a three-month-old may actually need a nap after only forty-five minutes of wakefulness. We will talk about awake span and how to tell if your baby is ready for a nap in Part II of this chapter.

Sleep and Feeding

Do formula-fed babies sleep better than breastfed ones? Does the introduction of solid foods improve sleep? It may surprise you, but the answer to both questions is no. It is absolutely true that babies have tiny tummies and need to eat frequently. It is also true that breastmilk is quicker to digest than formula and solid foods. Yet sleep and feeding are not as linked as it may seem. Breastfeeding has actually been shown to help young babies sleep *more* hours at night.[125] In older babies, breastfeeding is associated with more frequent night wakings,[113] but that may be because breastfeeding moms are more likely to respond quickly to a night waking, not because of the method of feeding itself.[95,134] In other words, breastfeeding moms more often create and support, intentionally or not, a feeding-to-sleep association, but it is absolutely possible to have a breastfed sound sleeper.

Introducing solid foods does not, on its own, help babies sleep better. Babies who receive more milk and solids during the day are less likely to *feed* at night, but are just as likely to *wake up*.[135]

Remember that babies' sleep cycles are only about forty minutes long and babies tend to wake up briefly as they transition between them?[81,92] A baby doesn't wake up *because* she's hungry; rather, she wakes up naturally between sleep cycles and *may or may not* be hungry. When a baby is used to eating at every awakening—because eating is her sleep association—she will call out every time. If, on the other hand, your baby knows how to go back to sleep on her own, she will go back to sleep *unless her need to eat is greater than her need to sleep.* When she is hungry, she will let you know, and you will not need to guess.

Sleep and Teething

Teething is a normal physiological process of the teeth moving in the jaw until they reach a baby's mouth. Contrary to popular belief,[136, 137] scientific studies have not found teething itself to cause fever, diarrhea, rashes, or sleep disruptions.[138-141] Because many babies show some of these symptoms around "tooth days," and because babies continue to get new teeth over many months starting around the middle of their first year, teething often becomes a scapegoat for any fussiness or sleep issues. If your baby has symptoms such as fever or loose stools, don't assume it's "just teething": see your baby's health care practitioner to rule out illness.

If your baby is healthy, teething is likely to make her gums only mildly sore, and only right around the time of the tooth emerging. If your baby generally settles to sleep on her own, this mild discomfort is unlikely to cause night wakings. It is also unlikely to require pain relief. Although teething gels are commonly suggested, several have been shown to have side effects.[137, 139, 142]

SLEEP FOUNDATION: KEY POINTS

- Sound sleep, just like healthy nutrition, gives babies a strong base upon which to grow.
- Baby's sleep structure develops by three to four months. After that there is no built-in biological improvement in baby's sleep.
- No one sleeps through the night: all of us, adults and babies alike, wake up briefly several times. To sleep soundly, a baby needs to smoothly transition between sleep cycles: go back to sleep calmly after waking unless she has a need greater than sleep.
- To smoothly transition between sleep cycles, babies must be well-rested. To stay well-rested, babies need a calm environment and a predictable daily rhythm, with an early bedtime and regular naps.
- To smoothly transition between sleep cycles, babies also need consistent sleep associations. They naturally look for patterns and sleep best when the same sleep cues are present at the beginning and in the middle of the night or a daytime nap.

Let's explore how we can set the stage for sound sleep in our homes.

PART II
A SLEEP-SUPPORTIVE ENVIRONMENT

With my first baby, as we went through many sleepless nights and no-good-nap days, I wondered: What can I do? What should I do? What am I doing wrong? I felt an immense sense of responsibility for her whole being and yet couldn't figure out just what to do to help her sleep better. Now, after navigating babyhood with my children and learning about the science behind sleep, I truly believe that our role is not to "train" or even teach our babies how to sleep. Neither do we have to wait out the first months or years. Rather, our role is to create environments conducive to sleep, build practices that support natural sleep development, and help babies see "this is how we sleep in our family."

Numerous books and online resources offer specific formulas for getting your baby to sleep. But the thing is, you cannot *make* your baby sleep: the act of falling asleep is something your baby has to do himself. You are responsible for the sleep environment and your baby decides whether and how much to sleep.

I would like to invite you to think about the knowledge discussed in Part I as you create the environment for sound sleep in your family. Regardless of where and how your baby sleeps, the three building blocks are: (1) a safe and soothing sleeping space, (2) responsive and consistent care, and (3) a balanced daily rhythm. You can add your personal perspective, cultural beliefs, and unique circumstances to these building blocks to create the sleep environment and sleep practices that work for you and your baby.

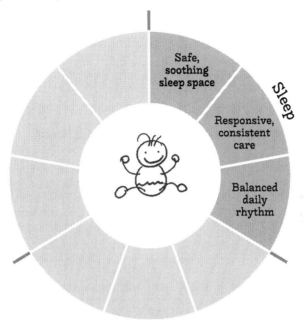

The ONE approach: Universal building blocks for sleep.

You may be awaiting your baby's arrival or your baby may already be here. In either case, you have your history, expectations, and beliefs around sleep, as well as your family's current sleep habits and needs to consider. Ask yourself the following questions. There are no right or wrong answers. Your answers may change in a few weeks or months, and that's okay. Answer as you see things today.

- What are my feelings around sleeping arrangements (bed-sharing, room-sharing, baby sleeping in her own room)? Where would I like my baby to sleep? Why?
- What do I imagine myself doing at bedtime and during night wakings when my baby is a newborn? A six-month-old? A twelve-month-old?

- What does being sensitive and responsive mean to me, in the context of sleep?
- What are my feelings and thoughts around crying?
- (If you have a partner) Are my partner and I on the same page when it comes to sleep in our family? If our perspectives differ, now or in the future, how will we manage disagreements?
- What are cultural practices and beliefs around babies' sleep in my extended family? Within my circle of friends? In my community?

Next, imagine what your daily rhythm, bedtimes, and nights with your baby will look like. Check your vision against three simple but important criteria:

1. Is it safe?
2. Does it feel respectful to my baby and true to my beliefs?
3. Is it consistent? Will it create a rhythm and help my baby see the patterns?

As you check your vision for consistency, think about it from your own perspective *and from your baby's perspective.*

Alyssa is expecting her first baby. She would like him to sleep in his own room. At bedtime, she imagines feeding and rocking him to sleep. She will respond as soon as her baby wakes up at night and nurse and rock him back to sleep. She will not leave him to cry. Alyssa hopes he will sleep through the night by nine months, the time she plans to return to work.

From Alyssa's perspective, this plan will allow her to spend special time with her baby and be consistent and responsive to his needs while preserving her adult time and space.

But let's look at this plan from the baby's perspective. He wakes up at night and finds himself in a very different environment from where he fell asleep: he was with Mommy and now is alone in his crib. Because he associates going to sleep with nursing and the sensation of being rocked, he may call out every time he awakens, whether he has a need greater than his need for sleep—for example, feeling hungry or wet—or he doesn't. By six months he will learn about patterns, establish associations, and likely call out every couple of hours, up from once or twice per night when he was a younger baby. He may continue calling out after he no longer needs night feedings.

This will involve Alyssa getting up several times every night, likely much past nine months, which may or may not work for her. As an alternative, Alyssa might want to explore safe bed-sharing to enjoy the closeness and to not have to get out of bed during night feedings so she can get more rest herself. Or she could consider a long nursing-and-rocking time in the morning—on the way out of, rather than into, sleep—and building a warm bedtime routine after which her baby is placed into his crib awake and goes to sleep on his own.

As you walk through your sleep vision with your baby's perspective in mind, see if you feel the need to adjust it. You can, of course, make changes later on when your baby is older. In fact, you can change your approach completely if you feel the need to. Making changes will take time and effort, but as long as your new vision is still safe and respectful, and supports consistency, it is absolutely okay to change course. What you wouldn't want to do is change course suddenly and reactively, out of one night's desperation and without preparing the space in advance, which we will talk about in the next section.

Keep your vision in mind as you work on the first building block of sound sleep: a safe and soothing space for sleep.

A safe and soothing space for sleep

Sleep arrangement and safety

Which sleeping arrangement fits most harmoniously with your family: bed-sharing, room-sharing, or baby sleeping in her own room? When you make your choice consciously, you will be able to create a sleeping space that puts your baby's safety first.

Bed-sharing

If you are considering bed-sharing, look for supportive, up-to-date education on how to practise it safely. Unlike cribs that are designed to meet safety standards for babies, adult beds are made for adult needs and comfort. Consider the room temperature, the design and position of the family bed, the bedding, and anything that may impair the responsiveness of the adults who bed-share with the baby. You should not bed-share if any of the following applies to your situation:

- You or your partner smoke
- You have consumed alcohol or taken any medication (legal or not) that may impair responsiveness
- You sleep on a sofa, air mattress, waterbed, or another soft surface
- You formula-feed
- Your baby was born pre-term
- You already bed-share with other children or pets
- You are severely fatigued

Find up-to-date recommendations on safe sleep by the American Academy of Pediatrics (AAP) or an equivalent organization in your country. Do talk to your baby's health care practitioner, even if you suspect they will strongly advise you against bed-sharing. If they do advise against it, consider this advice seriously; if you still feel that bed-sharing is the most harmonious choice for your family, find a health care practitioner or a professional organization that offers supportive and evidence-based advice on whether and how to practise bed-sharing safely in your particular situation. Take the time to think through and prepare the environment.

Room-sharing

If you are planning on room-sharing—having your baby sleep on her own sleep surface such as a crib or bassinet in your bedroom—you are not introducing the risks that bed-sharing may bring, yet still staying at arms reach. This is the safest and most recommended option.[111] However, room-sharing often brings the least amount of rest for parents. Parents are tuned into their babies and babies are noisy sleepers, so you may end up waking up with every little grunt, rustle, and snort. Think about how you'll get the rest you need—and with that, how you'll keep night feedings safe. If you're planning on feeding in a chair or sofa, take utmost care to not fall asleep during feedings. Chairs and sofas create extremely unsafe sleep environments for babies[111] because a baby can get wedged between the cushions or pressed against an armrest, all serious suffocation hazards. If you plan on bringing your baby into your bed for feedings, put the same consideration, thought, and careful planning into setting up your bed as you would for bed-sharing—in case you fall asleep while feeding.

Baby sleeping solo

If your baby is going to sleep in his own room, think about how you will make sure you hear him calling you at night. A variety of baby monitors are available on the market, some with not only sound, but also video and motion pad functions. You may find reassurance in having advanced functions or you may discover that less gives you more. Similar to the room-sharing scenario, you will need to think carefully about how to make feedings safe and not fall asleep while feeding in a chair or sofa. Don't bring your baby into bed with you out of one night's desperation, without addressing safety aspects beforehand.

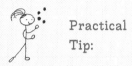

Practical Tip:

I used a clip-on night light with a built-in soft alarm during night feeds. I found it reassuring: if I did fall asleep, the alarm would wake me up after fifteen minutes, the usual length of our feedings.

I also thought of how I could make myself more comfortable. I knew that I needed to stay hydrated and have warm feet to return to sleep quickly once I was back in bed, so I kept a glass of water near my nursing chair and wore a pair of warm cozy socks when I got up to feed at night.

Regardless of the sleeping arrangement you decide on, remember these important sleep safety points:

- ✓ Choose a firm, natural sleeping surface
- ✓ Make sure no cords, strings, loose sheets, pillows, blankets, toys, or curtains are within baby's reach
- ✓ Always place baby to sleep on her back. At some point in the first year, your baby will start rolling onto her tummy by herself and may choose to sleep in this position. This is okay; there is no need to roll her back
- ✓ Be particularly careful when your baby is sleeping in an unfamiliar environment (for example, when travelling)

Do not plan to have your baby sleep in sitting devices like baby swings and rock-and-plays. These were not designed for sleeping, and sleeping in them can be unsafe. A baby sleeping in a sitting position can slump forward, which can restrict his airway and cause him to stop breathing; there's also a risk of being strangled by improperly secured straps. If you suspect your baby has reflux and could benefit from sleeping in a reclined position, raise this with your baby's health care practitioner and discuss the safest way to do it.

Babies, especially young ones, often fall asleep in their car seats. If your baby falls asleep in a car seat, keep an eye on him and take him out of the seat when you leave the vehicle. Don't bring the bucket-type car seat with you to let your baby continue napping. A recent study showed that of all babies who died sleeping in sitting devices, most died in car seats that were not being used as directed.[143] Removing the seat from its base and placing it on another surface can change the baby's recline and put him at risk for airway restriction. When my babies fell asleep in their car seats, I usually gently moved them into a crib; if I knew the nap was almost over and didn't want to disturb them, I stayed with them, watching carefully, in the car.

Sleeping space

After all safety aspects are covered, it is time to set up your baby's sleeping space. Choose non-toxic materials and natural, breathable fabrics, especially for the mattress, sheets, and sleepwear. After all, your baby will be spending more than half of her first year sleeping and her airway and delicate skin will be in contact with these materials. Natural fibres like 100% cotton breathe and regulate temperature better than synthetic materials. I don't find it's particularly useful to have a complete crib bedding set with a quilt, bumper pads, and crib skirt; in the first year, all you need is a firm, flat mattress tightly covered with a fitted sheet. Loose bedding and soft objects—blankets, pillows, bumper pads, and toys—are not safe because they can obstruct a baby's nose and mouth.[111]

If the temperature of your baby's sleeping space changes throughout the day and night, you might find it helpful to have a room thermometer to help you choose baby's sleepwear. Generally, it's best to keep baby's sleeping space cool. Although no specific temperature guidelines exist, the rule of thumb is that if the room is comfortable for you, it should be comfortable for your baby.[111, 144] For cozy, safe, and easy to put on sleepwear, consider one-piece cotton sleepers or onesies, with a baby sleep sack overtop. Sleep sacks usually come with a thermal property rating and a suggested room temperature range. If in doubt, go for under-dressing your baby: if she gets cold, she will wake up and let you know. An over-bundled baby, however, may not be awake enough to call out and may get overheated, which poses serious health risks.

Many websites and books recommend sound machines to mask the noise in baby's environment or to introduce soothing sounds. However, I would not put a sound machine on a list of must-haves. A recent study tested a sample of widely available models and found that all of them, when placed thirty centimetres away from the baby, were louder than the recommended noise level in hospital nurseries. Some machines even exceeded occupational limits for adults.[145] For families who choose to use a sound machine, the authors of this study suggest placing it as far away from the baby as possible (never on the crib rail) and playing the sound at a low volume and for a limited time. I would add that in most cases using a sound machine is unnecessary, as babies get accustomed to sleeping through the normal hum of their household. The sound of the machine can become one of baby's sleep associations and she may thus expect to hear it when she stirs in the middle of the night, leading you to have the sound on all night. That being said, advice on the other end of the spectrum, such as "save all your vacuuming for when your baby naps so he gets used to sleeping through anything" does not sit right with me either, because vacuuming when a family member is sleeping does not feel sensitive to me.

Keep baby's sleeping space dark at night to help him establish and maintain his circadian rhythm. Use blinds or blackout curtains and turn off all lights and screens. If you use a night light during feedings and diaper changes, choose a dim one, preferably with red or yellow light rather than white or blue. White and blue-based lights (including the illuminated screens of TVs, tablets, smartphones, and laptops) inhibit melatonin production and can thus disrupt the circadian rhythm by tricking the brain into thinking it is daytime.

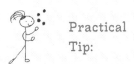

Practical
Tip:

Arrange nighttime diaper-change supplies next to where your baby sleeps, so you don't have to look for anything or carry your baby into another room in the middle of the night. You will need a waterproof pad, diapers, wipes, and a few changes of sleep clothes.

Finally, think of the overall feel of your baby's sleeping space. Does it feel calm or busy? Does it send the message to rest or to be active and play? Remember, baby does not need a particular colour scheme, a certain type of mobile, or any mobile at all: he will be just as interested in exploring his own hands, a pattern on the bed sheet, and the lines formed by the crib slats. But decorating the nursery or part of the room your baby will sleep in can be a special time for you. I remember sitting in a spot where we were planning on placing the crib just so I could get a sense of what my daughter would be able to see and hear from her vantage point.

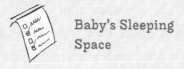

Baby's Sleeping Space

Must-haves:

- ✓ Caregiver nearby
- ✓ Firm, flat, natural sleeping surface
- ✓ Breathable sleepwear appropriate for room temperature
- ✓ Safe and comfortable place for night feedings

Good to have:

- ✓ Nighttime diaper-change supplies
- ✓ Room thermometer

Things to avoid:

- ✗ Pillows
- ✗ Toys near sleeping surface
- ✗ Bumper pads
- ✗ Overly loud sound machines

Responsive and consistent care

Join any local parenting group or online community and you'll soon find yourself amid a heated debate on the "right" approach to baby sleep. I never believed there was only one correct approach, and so when I first imagined this chapter, I planned to break it into two sections. One section, I thought, would focus on nighttime care suggestions for a family who wants their baby to sleep on her own. Another section would have advice for a family who would like to bed-share. But as I read through more and more research papers, I realized that from the sleep ecology perspective, there is no difference in the advice I would give. Both of these hypothetical families are already shaping their babies' sleep; both would benefit from babies falling asleep on their own; both need to focus on being responsive and consistent; and both need to be the timekeepers of their babies' daily rhythms. Let's take a closer look.

What you do matters

You are shaping your baby's sleep no matter what you do. Whether you actively soothe your baby to sleep or your baby goes to sleep on his own, he learns to recognize it as a pattern. Swaddling, rocking, nursing, pacifier, bottle, swing, car seat, Daddy's arms... through these experiences our babies learn how to go to sleep and return to sleep. Remember, genetics explains only about 50 percent of the differences in sleep patterns; caregiving shapes the other half.

I like to think of nighttime care as *sleep guiding*: we help baby see "this is how we sleep" while supporting his innate needs and abilities in a caring, loving, and responsive way. To me, being responsive does not necessarily mean responding right away, but rather learning to understand my baby and caringly responding to her needs. Many a time, it is one and the same thing: the pull to immediately pick up and soothe a crying baby is natural and strong. But sometimes I felt that my most caring response was to not pick my daughter up instantly, but to watch her closely to see what she was telling me; other times it involved not offering her a distraction, but hearing her cry in my arms. Responsive caregiving may mean something different to you. But as you respond, take a moment to quietly watch your baby and see what she's telling you.

Create consistency: sustainable sleep associations and routines

It is helpful to have consistent associations and warm, calm, and predictable routines around sleep. The best bedtime routines are formed together with our babies in response to their individual needs. For example, many families make a warm bath part of their baby's bedtime routine. However, if your baby finds having a bath stimulating rather than soothing, you may want to bathe him during the day instead.

Besides being consistent and soothing, your sleep routine must be *sustainable for you*. A sustainable routine is one you are able to do, keep up with, and enjoy every day. For example, bouncing your baby on an exercise ball may work for a while, but can soon become hard on your back and arms.

Next, think of whether your routine leads to *sustainable sleep associations for your baby*: will the conditions be generally the same at bedtime and when your baby wakes up at night?

A simple and soothing bedtime routine for ten-month-old Kylee, for example, includes quiet play time with Daddy followed by a bath, feeding, lights out, cuddle, and a song as Mommy places her into her crib before leaving the room. When Kylee wakes up in the middle of the night, the room is still dark, quiet, and the smells and feel of the space are the same as when she went to sleep; if she is hungry, she calls out, and if not, she goes back to sleep. Kylee's nap routine is a shorter version of the same general sequence: her nanny draws curtains in, gives her a hug, and sings a song.

Here's another example of a sustainable bedtime routine: Mommy goes to bed at night at the same time as six-month-old Declan. She nurses him to sleep in the family bed set up for safe bed-sharing and nurses him back to sleep during night wakings.

She carries him in a wrap during his morning nap and naps with him in the family bed in the afternoon.

Consistency is important, but it does not mean that the bedtime routine has to be done by the same adult every day or by one adult only. You may want to share the closeness of baby's bedtime with your partner (for example, one of you bathes the baby and the other puts him to bed), alternate days, or choose another arrangement that works for you. You and your partner may do things differently, but following the same general sequence at bedtime will help your baby recognize the familiar pattern. On days when a grandparent or a nanny is putting your baby to bed, having them follow your usual bedtime routine will help your baby settle for sleep easier.

Support self-settling

Remember, no baby truly sleeps through the night: all babies wake up, but some go back to sleep on their own as they transition between sleep cycles, without waking *us*. Because of this, there is no point in trying to prevent night wakings. Instead, we need to support our babies in returning to sleep after a waking, with or without our presence.

The term "self-soothing" holds a negative connotation to some people, as it seems to imply that instead of actively comforting an upset baby, the caregiver leaves the baby to his own devices. I wholeheartedly agree that babies should not be left to "self-soothe" from a place of distress. However, a baby who woke between sleep cycles may be tired, but not necessarily upset or in distress. Remember, most babies make at least brief attempts to return to sleep on their own when they wake up.[95] When a baby goes to sleep calmly on his own, I think of it as *baby's own self-settling routine*. When a baby is tended to by a parent during a night waking, I think of it as a *parent and baby's interaction and re-settling routine*. In both cases, the relaxing and going to sleep is always done by babies themselves, as this is something we simply cannot do for them.

Do you want your baby to self-settle? I think most, if not all, parents do, regardless of their sleep arrangement. Whether your baby sleeps with you or on his own, his ability to self-settle during those wakings when he is comfortable, but still tired and in need of more sleep, is what will bring more sound sleep to both of you. It will also bring you peace of mind. When you know your baby is capable of self-settling and you hear him calling out, you won't have to lie in bed listening and guessing whether you should go to him. If he calls out, you know he likely has a *need greater than his need for sleep*. Finally, if your baby knows how to self-settle, when he gets to the point where he is no longer hungry at night, he will "sleep through."

To prepare for sleeping long stretches down the road, you can begin guiding your baby toward self-settling in the early months. As often as possible, give your baby opportunities to experience what it feels like to go to sleep on her own. When she wakes up after a short nap, leave her for a few minutes to see if she goes back to sleep. Another good opportunity is putting your baby to bed while she is awake. Many books and online resources recommend putting baby to bed "drowsy but awake." The problem is that most parents don't have a good idea of what "drowsy but awake" looks like and tend to wait until baby is almost asleep before placing her into the crib. This can feel jarring, and baby will likely startle or protest, especially if she is older than a few weeks. Instead, try putting your baby to bed tired, but *completely awake*. A good time to try this is after a relaxing bedtime routine on a day your baby had good naps and is settled and well-rested overall.

Instead of looking for "drowsy but awake" signs, try putting your baby to bed tired but completely awake to let her practise self-settling.

Let's look at the third (and final) building block of sound sleep: a balanced, age-appropriate daily rhythm.

A balanced daily rhythm

Help your baby stay well-rested by creating a predictable rhythm to her days, with regular nap opportunities and early bedtimes. Without that, baby's internal rhythms—those created by the homeostatic, circadian, and ultradian drives—won't work in harmony. If a baby sometimes goes to bed at 9 p.m. and other times at 6 p.m., when she's in bed at 6 p.m. her body doesn't know whether to expect a late nap or an early bedtime and whether she should sleep one hour or eleven. Her sleep structure becomes disorganized.[121]

From Your Baby's
Perspective:

Imagine taking a transatlantic flight and arriving at your destination early in the morning. You might decide to take a nap or push through till the evening to adjust to the local time. Now imagine that you don't know what local time is, when and if you're taking your next flight, and when you'll have a chance to rest properly again. How will you know whether and for how long to sleep for?

This is how a baby who misses a nap might feel. Naps structure a baby's day into little windows of awake time in the same way nights divide weeks into days for older children and adults. A baby who normally naps every hour and a half, but stays up for three hours, may feel the same as an adult who got up on Monday morning and didn't get to sleep again until Tuesday night!

Build your days at home with your baby around her naps. Plan to give your baby opportunities to have most of her naps and night sleep in her usual space. Think of naps not as isolated time periods, but rather as part of a daily rhythm, in which each sleep period influences the others. Be the timekeeper: protect your baby's sleep structure and daily rhythm. That way, occasional "different days" when you are out and about, or when a nap just doesn't happen, shouldn't be a problem.

Catch the developmental wave: a stage-by-stage guide

Let's now put everything together to help your baby develop a natural sleep pattern and get the sleep she needs, adjusting as she grows. When you read about the different ages and stages, here and elsewhere, try not to get overwhelmed by the average time-lines and milestones. Rather, use them as guideposts in getting to know your own unique baby. Sound sleep is not a finish line, but an unfolding process.

Birth to 6 weeks

- *For baby: Focus on feeding, soothing, and getting to know your baby.*
- *For you: Focus on rest, healing, and getting to know yourself as a parent (or reflecting on your parenting journey so far).*

In these early weeks, your baby will often fall asleep while feeding, snuggled in your arms, or carried in a baby carrier. When he does, enjoy the snuggles, the little head on your chest, and the new baby smell. Some naps will be long and some short. Don't worry about the clock. Follow your baby's need for rest and look for opportunities to rest yourself.

When your baby is sleeping in your arms and you want to place him in a crib or bassinet, wait at least ten minutes from the time he falls asleep to make sure he's in deep (non-REM) sleep. If one day your baby doesn't fall asleep after a feeding and looks calm and content, try laying him down in his sleeping space and watch quietly. He may look around for a bit and go to sleep on his own. If he doesn't, try again another time. Don't worry about consistency yet and don't have any expectations; simply offer your baby these brief opportunities for going to sleep on his own as they happen, every now and then.

Your baby may sleep more during the day than at night or take brief naps around the clock. Remember that this is a short and special stage: the day-night confusion will end when your baby begins making enough melatonin to develop a clear circadian rhythm. To help this rhythm emerge, bring in natural light during the day. Spend time outdoors if you can: a blanket on a shaded balcony or under a tree in a backyard are wonderful, simple options. During night feedings and diaper changes, keep the light dim and stimulation low, making the room dark and calm. I encourage you not to turn on the TV or other screens and stick to "night mode," even when your baby is awake for longer periods of time. You could hold her, cuddle her, nurse her just for comfort, sing softly, walk with her or place her beside you and watch her quietly. Experiment to see what brings your baby most contentment and helps her go back to sleep. If you're breastfeeding, the melatonin in your milk will help your baby sleep at night. (However, if you feed your baby expressed milk, remember that if it was expressed during the day it won't have much melatonin, which is only detectable in nighttime breastmilk.[126]) Your gentle support will help your baby's internal sleep rhythms develop and will eventually lead to longer stretches of sleep for both of you.

The total amount of time babies sleep in twenty-four hours ranges widely at this stage, from nine to nineteen hours. Most babies sleep somewhere between thirteen and sixteen hours a day.[96] Many go to sleep easily at this stage, but some—about one in five—do not.

If your baby doesn't go to sleep easily and is agitated or crying a lot when awake, please remember, first and foremost, that this is:

- Not a predictor of your baby's personality or future sleep patterns[146]
- Not something that will last forever
- Not your fault

Your baby's behaviour may or may not fit the classic definition of colic. Colic usually starts a few days after birth (or after the original due date for premature babies), peaks at six weeks, and disappears by three or four months. Long crying and fussing spells happen mostly in the evenings.

Remember that all babies are irritable, fuss, and cry some of the time. Colic is a more-than-average amount of this normally occurring fussiness—one end of the continuum between a very settled and a very unsettled baby. Colic is not something a baby *has*. Think of it as something he *does*—the way he expresses himself during these early weeks when the world probably feels very big and overwhelming to him.

How can you best help your unsettled baby? We know that being tired exacerbates colic, and that colicky babies have a harder time feeling rested because they sleep less[30, 121] and become overtired more easily. Try to keep your baby as calm and rested as possible. Keep stimulation low and experiment with soothing: creating gentle motion, going outside, comfort nursing, holding her upright against your body, carrying her in a wrap, playing soft music, or placing her on her back on a blanket on the floor with you nearby. Plan for extra-long soothing during the evening hours, especially at around six weeks.

If your baby is unsettled, you may be feeling tired, sad, helpless, overwhelmed, or angry. These feelings can be scary, but please know that they are normal. It's also essential to ask for help when you need it. Help may come in the form of a long phone call with a friend across the continent who's been through it (with both of her kids, even though she thought lightning surely wouldn't strike twice; they all survived and her kids are great!). Help may come in the form of your partner or a close family member reliably taking care of your baby for a certain amount of time each day, so you can experience some quiet and stillness: a hot shower, a bowl of soup, a nap, or something else that makes you feel cared for.

If, on the other hand, your baby goes to sleep easily and sleeps a lot, and you're feeling well, it might seem reasonable and convenient to have your baby nap on the go as you shop, run errands, or visit family and friends. But if you were my sister, I would urge you to stay close to home most days during the first few weeks, for three important reasons.

The first reason is your own rest and healing. Your mind and body need time to adjust and recover. As much as you may want to get back on your feet and "get things done," wait. Remember the postpartum "babymoon" or "bubble" practice I mentioned in Chapter 1? Try to create your own version of a postpartum bubble, if only for a short while.

The second reason to stay close to home during the first few weeks is that a baby who mostly sleeps on the go may get overstimulated and very tired. Some babies do sleep well in busy environments during the early weeks, but others escape into sleep as a way to tune out overstimulation.[128] These babies are not getting the deep sleep they need at the time they need it. As days go by, they may get tired and become difficult to soothe. Studies have shown that among babies four months and older who are described as "difficult sleepers," almost half had no trouble sleeping in the early weeks.[121] It could be that these babies were the very "portable" ones who ended up overstimulated and overtired.

The third reason to stay close to home is this: the early weeks are a once-in-a-lifetime opportunity to gently welcome your baby into the world and to get to know him and his sleep needs. Watch your baby nap: does he make noises in his sleep? Try to figure out his sleeping sounds and how they differ from his "I-am-awake-and-need-you" sounds. This knowledge will be very helpful when your baby begins linking sleep cycles into longer stretches of sleep. When you hear something that sounds like his sleepy noises, you will know not to pick him up —you don't want to wake a sleeping baby.

Watch your baby to see what he finds soothing and what makes him more awake and alert. Does a bath relax him and help him fall asleep or does it make him more active? During a middle-of-the-night diaper change, does it matter whether the wipe is warm or cold? What does your baby do just before he goes to sleep? Can you see signs of tiredness? Parenting resources often suggest looking for sleep cues like eye rubbing, ear pulling, and yawning. But in my experience, these, along with fussiness, are signs of an *over*tired baby. Instead, look for the slight quieting, staring off, calmness, a lull in energy. If you don't notice any particular tired signs yet, don't worry: just keep watching and getting to know your baby.

6 weeks to 3 months

- *For baby:* Focus on moving toward consistency, routines, and early bedtimes.
- *For you:* Use the emerging daily rhythm to make your time at home with your baby easier and more enjoyable.

At some point after the first six weeks you'll notice that your baby is generally sleeping for longer stretches at night than during the day and that her night wakings are getting shorter. These are signs of sleep consolidation. After sleep consolidation begins, a fairly consistent bedtime will start to emerge. Initially it will be late, often between 10 p.m. and midnight, but it will gradually shift to an earlier time over the following few weeks. Your baby's longest stretch of night sleep will likely be the first one after she goes to bed. Try to catch some rest yourself before the first night feeding.

Now is a good time to think about a bedtime routine and to introduce some of its elements. Remember, the bedtime routine you create ultimately needs to be sustainable for you and bring sustainable sleep associations for your baby. For example, you may want to bathe your baby, dress him in a fresh diaper and sleepwear, sing a lullaby, and then feed him in his sleeping space, with the lights off. Talk to him softly, explaining what you're about to do as you move through each step of the routine together.

As your baby approaches three months, move toward consistency in where your baby naps and how you soothe him to sleep. Your nap routine can be the same as your bedtime routine, a shorter version of it, or it can be quite different. What matters is general consistency from day to day, enough for your baby to recognize familiar patterns.

Feeding can be a wonderful and natural part of your nap routine. As before, if your baby usually falls asleep in your arms during a feeding and naps separately from you, wait at least ten minutes before you move him to a crib or bassinet; remember, babies of this age don't enter deep sleep right away. Most babies need to be burped after each feeding at this age. Carrying your baby upright against your body or patting her back before you lay her down will help her burp and then nap more comfortably.

Your baby's naps are likely not yet regular: some may be short and some long, and the number probably still varies from day to day. Your baby is more alert than in the early weeks. Now is a good time to begin figuring out his optimal awake window: the best spacing between naps. Knowing this window will help you guide your baby toward sleep when his need to sleep (his homeostatic drive) has built up sufficiently, but overtiredness has not yet set in. As Dr. Marc Weissbluth says in *Healthy Sleep Habits, Happy Child*, "catch this wave of tiredness... you have to catch the wave after it rises enough to be recognized but before it crashes."[121] Your baby's *longest* awake window will almost never be longer than two hours at this stage, and in fact it could be as short as thirty minutes (really, that short!). His tired signs will appear before the end of his awake window. Look for that slight quieting, staring off, a lull in energy.

Practical Tip:

Keep notes on the timing of your baby's naps and bedtime to see if a pattern emerges. Do it consistently for at least two weeks. There are a number of websites and apps available to help you, but a simple pen-and-paper method works well too.

If you can't figure out the tired signs, don't worry and keep observing: you will have many more opportunities to see how your baby acts when he's tired! Try to pinpoint the overtired signs, think about how much time has passed since your baby's last nap, and work backward. If in doubt, try a shorter awake window.

Begin winding your baby down for a nap well *before* the end of the optimal awake window. For example, if you find that your baby comfortably stays awake for an hour, begin soothing her to sleep after forty-five to fifty minutes.

In the evening, start your bedtime routine at least half an hour before the end of your baby's awake window—and well before she begins looking or acting tired. At this stage, bedtime will vary from day to day, depending on when she woke from her last nap and how rested she is, but, as I mentioned, you will see bedtime gradually shift to an earlier hour. If you are not seeing this shift at all, think about your baby's last nap of the day. Sometimes what looks like a late nap is actually baby's natural bedtime. If you think this might be the case, try soothing your baby back to sleep after she wakes up from that late "nap." If she goes right back to sleep, she's telling you she's ready for an earlier bedtime.

Your baby's natural bedtime may shift to as early as 6:30 or 7 p.m. by about three months. This early bedtime means more restorative night sleep for your baby: ten or even twelve hours with night feedings in between. If your baby sleeps separately from you, you will now start getting more grown-up time in the evenings. However, you may also get less sleep because your baby's longest sleep stretch—the first one after she goes to bed—is no longer aligned with your own sleep. Adjust your own routines and go to bed early if you can.

You may feel as if between feeding and soothing your baby to sleep there is little time left for playing with her or showing her the world. Don't worry: soon her awake windows will lengthen naturally. For now, these short intervals of wakefulness are keeping your baby rested as you build, together, the foundation for sound sleep. And you are indeed building it together. As you soothe your baby to sleep, she's interacting with you, bonding, and learning, and the process of learning continues even as she sleeps. Flexible routines and a predictable rhythm create a flow from morning to noon to night for your baby and for your family as a whole. In our busy world, your baby needs you to notice the signs, help create the rhythm, and, as Karen Maezen Miller says in *Momma Zen*, "be the timekeeper."[147]

3 to 5 months

- *For baby: Support baby's emerging daily rhythm with regular naps and an early bedtime.*
- *For you: Remember to care for and nourish yourself.*

Once your baby's bedtime moves to an earlier hour and becomes more consistent, he will begin waking up for the day at a more consistent time, likely between 6 and 8 a.m. His awake windows will still be short, so he will be ready for his first nap only two hours or less (possibly much less) after getting up for the day. As his morning wake-up time becomes more consistent, so will the timing of the first nap. To give you an idea, many babies go down for their first nap between 8 and 9 a.m. at this stage. Take note of the timing of the morning nap, but watch your baby and his tired signs—he's still your best guide.

A day in the life of a three-month-old baby might look like this:

A Four-Nap Day
7:00 a.m.: wake up
8:00–9:00 a.m.: first nap
10:30–11:30 a.m.: second nap
1:15–2:00 p.m.: third nap

4:00–4:30 p.m.: fourth nap
7:00 p.m.: asleep for the night

If feeding is part of your baby's nap routine and he naps separately from you, by this point he may no longer be falling asleep in your arms after a feeding. It is easy to take that as a sign that he should stay awake longer, but that's usually not the case. He is simply more alert now and his sleep structure is changing. Try putting your baby to bed awake after a feeding and see if he goes to sleep on his own. I don't recommend waiting for your baby to be in the twilight zone of "almost asleep" before putting him down: there is a good chance he will startle and, understandably, become upset. I believe that giving him the chance to practise solo sleep from a place of being tired, but awake and content, is the most gentle and respectful way.

By about four months, your baby may get into a pattern of three naps a day, with the second nap after lunch and a third in mid-afternoon. His longest awake period will likely be one between his last nap of the day and bedtime,[80] for example:

A Three-Nap Day
7:00 a.m.: wake up
8:15–9:45 a.m.: first nap
11:30 a.m.–1:30 p.m.: second nap
3:30–4:15 p.m.: third nap
6:30 p.m.: asleep for the night

This is just an example to give you an idea of what a day *might* look like. Being aware of your baby's emerging rhythm will help you create the environment for him to sleep at predictable times, but don't feel as if you should get him on a schedule. If your baby's naps are mostly short, he may still take four naps some days (or even most days.) Keep watching for your baby's tired signs and adjusting your day following his lead.

As your baby moves toward three naps a day, it's important to keep the early bedtime. There may be days when you cannot fit a fourth nap in, but three naps are not quite enough. On those days, go through your usual bedtime routine, but start it an hour or so earlier.

Does this sound like a lot of careful observation and adjustment? Well, it is. More predictable days are just around the corner. For now it is important to help your baby stay as well-rested as possible to support the development of his sleep structure.

Now, you might have heard of something that happens around four months: the dreaded four-month sleep regression. Many families comment that their previously good sleeper began waking frequently at night and "refusing" naps at this age. Approximately 9 percent of babies have a very hard time sleeping at this age; some of these babies had colic and some did not.[121] Many other babies still sleep fairly well, but wake up more than they did before. What is going on?

First, remember the changes in baby's sleep structure that happen around four months? Your baby's sleep is becoming more adult-like. She is developing distinct sleep cycles and tends to wake up briefly after each period of REM sleep. In a sense, this is a *progression* rather than a regression. I think of it as a sleep shift.

Second, there are many developmental leaps happening around this age: your baby is learning to roll, grasp, and use her voice in different ways; she's growing fast. She is working hard and may need extra time to wind down.

Finally, if a baby has not been getting the rest she needs in the early weeks, overtiredness may be catching up to her. She may have been going to bed too late, mostly sleeping on the go, or staying awake too long between naps. As she moves to three naps a day, she may become overtired and her sleep may get disorganized.

If you feel your baby is overtired, think about how you can offer her more sleep. Can you move her bedtime to an earlier hour or shorten her awake times? Might your baby be getting overstimulated when she's awake and, because of that, having a harder time winding down? Can you make changes to her sleeping space to make it more conducive to sleep (for example, making it darker, quieter, or cooler)?

Even if your baby is well-rested, he's still going through the sleep shift and developmental leaps, so there's a good chance you'll notice at least some signs of sleep regression. To help your baby navigate this phase, put extra effort into keeping him well-rested. Continue to carefully watch his awake windows; if in doubt, put him to bed earlier. Continue offering your baby naps in his usual sleeping space and the comfort of familiar routines. For a baby who had colic, expect to put in an even greater effort in being regular and consistent to help him stay calm and rested.

Many sleep experts recommend beginning some form of sleep training around this age, which usually involves cutting out at least some nighttime feeds. I disagree with this approach. Continue feeding your baby when he's hungry. Don't introduce solid foods before four months in hopes of getting more sleep. Remember, your baby doesn't wake up *because* he's hungry; rather, he wakes up naturally between sleep cycles.

It's also important to resist reverting to the late bedtime your baby had when she was younger. Sometimes parents go back to a late bedtime because their baby seemed to sleep better that way. The thing is, it's *parents* who were getting more sleep: the long stretch of baby's sleep—the first one after baby goes to bed—used to overlap with theirs. But as you may recall, a baby who goes to bed late gets less sleep overall[97,120] and can become overtired, which eventually leads to less sleep for the whole family.

You may be surprised by just how tired you are these days. The really early weeks are behind you, and you may have expected to have more energy or to be out and about more by now. But remember, you are still healing and adjusting emotionally and physically and probably have not had many (or any) full nights of sleep yet. To help yourself stay better rested, think about how you can work more sleep into your day. Sleep when baby sleeps (if you can). If you're bed-sharing, consider napping with your baby or going to bed at the same time as your baby in the evening.* If you can't sleep when baby sleeps, try to at least incorporate more *rest* into your day or things that fill your cup: a walk outside, a book, a nourishing meal. Try not to focus on tiredness in a negative way or wish you could be more active or productive. In Karen Maezen Miller's words, "Don't reject it… don't inflate it with meaning or difficulty. Be what you are: be tired."[147]

5 to 6 months

- *For baby: Protect daily rhythm, support longer naps.*
- *For you: Think about how little time has passed and how much has happened since your baby was born.*

Your baby has likely developed a somewhat predictable daily rhythm, with a fairly consistent morning wake-up time, daytime naps, and bedtime. She is hopefully sleeping more soundly now than during the sleep regression. Continue being the timekeeper to help her stay rested.

---

* If you plan on bed-sharing and putting your baby to sleep in a family bed before you go to bed yourself, make sure you very carefully assess your baby's safety. Consider putting your baby to sleep in a crib for the early part of the night and moving him in with you when you go to bed.

Your baby is learning or has recently mastered how to roll onto her tummy and may even be starting to crawl. She will likely practice this newfound mobility in her sleep and when she wakes up at night. She might roll over, get stuck, and call out for you, possibly many times a night. To encourage this short phase to pass, give your baby the space and time to practice free movement during the day while you watch quietly nearby. She may grunt as she struggles to master a new skill, but don't "rescue" her unless she's upset or has moved into an unsafe position. Once she's able to roll onto her tummy and is comfortable in that position, she might choose to sleep this way; many babies do. There's no need to roll her back over.

Your baby may also be cutting her first teeth around this time. Remember that teething is making her gums only mildly sore, and only right around the time each tooth emerges. Teething itself is unlikely to cause night wakings. Your baby may need extra soothing before naps and at bedtime, but other than that your routines can remain the same.

If, however, your baby has a fever, a rash, a runny nose, or is unusually irritable, don't just chalk it up to teething. Teething normally does not cause fevers, but colds and other illnesses do. As your baby becomes mobile, she is getting more opportunities to explore the world by mouthing objects. She is also likely spending more time outside the home, with you or in daycare, and is thus more likely to catch a virus. Watch her carefully for signs of illness and contact her health care practitioner if you're concerned.

How are your baby's naps? Her awake windows are likely still short, somewhere around two hours. If she used to take brief naps, there's a good chance they are getting longer now. If her naps are still more of a short "naplet"[89]—forty minutes or less—think about what you can do to help lengthen them. Continue to plan most of your baby's naps in her usual sleeping space. If you bed-share, see if you can soothe her back to sleep after a short nap by nursing, patting her back, or whatever you normally do to help her drift off to sleep. For a baby who sleeps separately from you, try one of these options:

- If you normally stay with her as she goes to sleep, go in right away and try to soothe her back to sleep.
- If she normally goes to sleep on her own, pause for a few minutes before going in when you first hear her: she might be just calling out in her sleep, or she might be awake but still tired and ready to go back to sleep.

Continue offering your baby opportunities to take longer naps, but when naps are short, don't worry: go for extra soothing and an earlier bedtime.

Many babies at this age are beginning to show interest in solid foods. Introducing your little one to the world of textures, aromas, and flavours is a special and exciting time. We will go over the signs of readiness and how to begin offering first foods in Chapter 3. For now, remember that introducing solids is unlikely to bring longer stretches of sleep, so don't rush it for that reason. Wait till your baby is ready, take it slow, and enjoy the start of this new phase that will last a lifetime: your child joining you at the family table.

6 to 8 months

- **For baby:** *Support the transition to two naps, and shift bedtime when needed.*
- **For you:** *Shift your bedtime to an earlier hour, too.*

Both your baby's naps and his time awake between naps are lengthening, and he's getting ready to move to napping just twice a day. For most babies this transition happens between six and eight months. The transition will begin all on its own; you'll just notice that there are suddenly days with no time left for a third nap. For example, if your baby doesn't get up from his second nap until 3 p.m., encouraging him to take a third nap at 5 p.m. would shift his bedtime to a late hour. Instead, skip the third nap and move his bedtime earlier. Look for tired signs, but generally aim for an awake span of three hours or less after the second nap of the day.

A seven-month-old baby's day might look like this:

A Two-Nap Day
6:45 a.m.: wake up
8:45–10:05 a.m.: first nap
1:00–3:00 p.m.: second nap
7:00 p.m.: asleep for the night

Again, this is just an example. If your baby's naps are short, he may take three naps on some days or even on most days. Remain consistent with where your baby sleeps and with your routines, but be flexible with bedtime timing: adjust it depending on how many naps your baby takes on any given day and how rested he is.

During the three-to-two naps transition, it is best to avoid brief snoozes in the car or stroller in the late afternoon and early evening. A ten-minute snooze is not enough for your baby to rest and replenish, but is enough to relieve his pressure to sleep (homeostatic sleep drive), which can make it harder for him to go to sleep at night. An occasional car trip in late afternoon is fine, of course, but try not to get into a pattern of two naps + mini-snooze = late bedtime. This pattern creates unbalanced sleep rhythms and can make the upcoming nine-month sleep regression more challenging.

8 to 10 months

- *For baby: Continue offering the comfort of familiar routines; talk to her if she protests sleep.*
- *For you: Enjoy more predictability during your days at home with your baby.*

Many parents notice a sleep regression at eight or nine months.[87] What is happening this time? It could be one or more of the following things.

First, your baby's working hard and once again may need extra time to wind down. She's going through many developmental leaps: learning to crawl, stand and perhaps even walk; trying a variety of foods; rapidly expanding her repertoire of sounds; putting things together and figuring out sequences. She may be practising her newfound skills—standing, for example—when she wakes up at night or even in her sleep. Put extra care into making sure she can't fall out of her crib or bed.

Second, your baby is beginning to understand complex sequences and not only see that certain events tend to follow one another, but also realize that *he* can make things happen (for example, he can put one block on top of another—or call Mommy and make her appear!). If your baby sleeps separately from you and is used to drifting off to sleep calmly on his own, he may now protest when you leave the room. This can stretch his bedtime well past the usual hour.

Finally, if your baby has not been getting enough rest lately, overtiredness may once again be catching up to him. He may have been going to bed too late or sleeping on the go. Now that he has moved to two naps a day, he could be overtired.

To help your baby navigate this phase, put extra effort into keeping him well-rested. Continue offering naps in his usual sleeping space and minimize mini-snoozes in the car or stroller.

Continue providing the comfort of familiar routines. At this age, the routines are still important for keeping your baby well-rested, but are also becoming extra helpful in guiding him toward understanding "this is how we sleep in our family":

- If you bed-share and it now takes a while for your baby to wind down at night, begin your routine a little earlier to keep the early bedtime.

- If your baby sleeps solo and usually self-settles, but now protests as you leave, talk to him. Acknowledge his feelings ("I see you would like me to stay"), tell him what you are going to do and let him know you will be near ("It's time for you to rest. I'm going to tidy up the kitchen and go to bed myself. I will be nearby if you need me"). Then leave, and come back if he calls to reassure and comfort him if he cries. You may need to go in several times, so start bedtime earlier if you can. Remember, this shift is happening because of your baby's new level of understanding of his environment. Similar to his new level of mobility, this is progress, a step forward.

- If your baby sleeps solo and you stay with him as he falls asleep, he may now be taking much longer to wind down. Is he acting as if he'd rather play than sleep? Tell him it's time to rest and continue with your usual routine; don't turn on the lights or take him out of his sleeping space. Remain consistent; he may go back to drifting off to sleep in your presence within a couple of weeks. If that doesn't happen, it's possible that your presence now feels more exciting than calming to him. Consider shifting toward having your baby self-settle for sleep—now is a good time. Explain the changes to your baby, go slow, and be consistent (for more advice on making changes, see pages 92–98).

Is your baby napping predictably twice a day now? If so, you can "lock naps in" and begin your nap routine at approximately the same time each day. This will bring more predictability to your day, making it easier to plan meals, walks, errands, and visits. Many babies begin their first nap around 9 a.m. and their second nap around 1 p.m. at this stage; however, choose nap times that work best for your baby.

10 to 12 months (and beyond)

- **For baby:** *Keep the afternoon nap.*
- **For you:** *Enjoy more flexibility during your days at home with your baby.*

If you remained consistent with your approaches, there is a good chance your baby is sleeping long stretches now. She may or may not be feeding at night, but if she does, she probably goes back to sleep quickly and easily.

If your baby is staying home with you, you might start thinking of transitioning her to one nap, so that you can spend more time out and about or to match an older sibling's rest time. Or your baby might be starting daycare or moving to an older-baby room at the daycare centre. Many daycares encourage older babies to nap once a day so they can join the routines and activities of toddlers. However, your baby is unlikely to be truly ready for the two-to-one-nap transition until she is around eighteen months old. Talk to your daycare provider to explore the option of keeping both naps for your baby for as long as she needs it.

That being said, you can now have occasional one-nap days: just plan for an earlier bedtime to keep your baby rested. This will bring more flexibility to your days and make it easier to plan outings and trips.

I would love to send you off with sleep advice that stretches beyond the first twelve months, but honestly, there isn't much more to say. As your baby grows, continue checking in with yourself to make sure the sleep environment is working for you, and continue observing your now-toddler, to make sure the sleep environment is working for her. Continue helping her stay rested. Tell her about and prepare her for any changes you may be introducing. And remember the foundation of sound sleep you have built together.

Sleep stories

An easy baby: Mason's sleep story

When other parents shared their sleep challenges at a local baby group, Sarah didn't know what to say: three-month-old Mason slept great. He was such a happy baby that she and Rick joked they must have won the Easy Baby Lottery. Mason's birth went smoothly, and he was feeding like a champ. Soon after coming home from the hospital, Sarah and Rick felt as if they jumped right back into their old life: just as before, they were always on the go, but now with their beautiful baby. Mason happily gazed at the world from his car seat, his stroller, or his parents' arms. He napped easily about every other hour; he was sometimes asleep, sometimes awake, and always content. At night, Sarah fed him to sleep while catching a late show and then gently transferred him into a bassinet near her side of the bed; Mason usually slept a good six-hour stretch, fed, and went right back to sleep for another two or three hours.

At around four and a half months, Mason began napping less. He still fell asleep easily in his car seat, but only napped for about twenty minutes. He now struggled to fall asleep at bedtime and stayed up after the evening feeding, often well past midnight. Sarah moved the glider into the living room and began rocking him to sleep. But Mason was now waking more at night: first twice, then three times, then four. Having him sleep in a swing by the bed helped some nights, but not always. Sarah began bringing Mason into bed with her to get some rest. She was tired, but remained hopeful that this stage would pass soon.

By six months Mason had a pretty consistent sleep pattern: he went to bed around 10 p.m., woke three to five times a night, and got up for the day around 5:30 a.m. He was now sleeping in a crib in his own room. Sarah fed and rocked him back to sleep, but the soothing was taking longer and longer. "He must be teething," reasoned Rick. After consulting with their pediatrician, Sarah and Rick began giving Mason infant pain-relief medicine before bed, yet that didn't bring relief. Sarah scoured the web for sleep-training advice, but none of the suggested methods seemed right. Instead, Rick took over two of the night feedings so Sarah could get more rest.

At eleven months, Mason was down to one short nap per day, which usually happened in the late afternoon in the car, and he still woke multiple times at night. Exhausted and desperate, Sarah and Rick decided to try the cry-it-out sleep-training approach called "extinction." Mason cried with such intensity that they changed their mind and went in after seven minutes—minutes that felt like eternity. They tried again at sixteen months; the first night Mason fussed for forty minutes, went to sleep on his own and only woke once, but during the second night he cried so hard they brought him into their bed.

Mason is now two and a half. He still naps at daycare during the week, but on weekends he only occasionally catches a mini-snooze in the car. When he does have a nap, his bedtime stretches well past 10 p.m.; he falls asleep with a tablet as it seems to be the only way to keep him in his bed. Most nights he is up a few times and eventually comes into Sarah and Rick's bed. Regardless of when he goes to sleep, Mason always wakes up for the day around 5:30 a.m. Sarah has read about the use of artificial melatonin for older children, but she's really hoping to not have to resort to it. Mason's baby sister is due to arrive any day now. Sarah and Rick joke that the transition to two kids should be super easy, as they are already as tired as they can possibly be... But sometimes they wonder: "What if we get another bad sleeper?"

By the book: Leah's sleep story

My firstborn's big dark eyes scanned the delivery room. "She's so alert for a newborn... she's taking it all in..." said the nurse. And so began our long journey to finding sleep.

I thought I was prepared. Before Leah was born, both Jason and I read a highly recommended book on infant sleep. I read three other books, just in case. I kept sleep and feeding records, and because of that I can tell you exactly how it all unfolded.

For the first couple of weeks Leah would fall asleep nursing, nap a solid two- or three-hour stretch, and then stay awake for about an hour at a time. I sometimes held her through her naps and sometimes placed her into her crib once she was asleep. At night she slept in a small room adjoining our bedroom; when she stirred, I nursed her, and she either went right back to sleep or stayed awake and calm while I held her for an hour or so.

At around two weeks old, Leah began having what we called "the evening fussies": she was wakeful and irritable between 5 and 10 p.m., but didn't sleep. We held her and I comfort-nursed her through those evenings.

By six weeks Leah's night sleep consolidated into a stretch from 10 p.m. to 8 a.m., with two or three feedings in between. But her naps grew short, mostly lasting forty minutes, and she *stopped falling asleep after nursing. In fact, after a while she stopped going down for a nap at all. Everyone who met her commented on just how alert she was: this baby sure didn't want to miss anything! Okay, I thought, this must be the time to begin putting her down drowsy but awake, as the books suggested. Trouble was, I didn't see any drowsy signs at all. Leah was alert and easily startled, but seemed active and happy all day long. The sleep programs recommended two-hour windows between naps, and so I began nursing Leah and putting her in the crib every two hours. But that didn't work. She called out as soon as I left the room. I came back, nursed or held her, and eventually she'd go to sleep, but she only ever slept for twenty to forty minutes. I tried pacifiers and swaddling, but neither made a difference. I felt as if I were spending my whole day trying for a nap, but she still slept very little, and we were both exhausted. Leah went to sleep easily on her own around 9 p.m. after our bedtime routine, but started waking more and more through the night. At four and a half months she began waking every hour; I nursed her every time. One night I literally walked into the wall, disoriented from fatigue.*

One night when Leah was six months old, I heard her calling. Just as I was about to pick her up to feed her, I noticed she was actually asleep. What if I'd been waking her by rushing in? I began waiting a few minutes before going in, both at night and when she woke up from napping. And she often went back to sleep; if she began to call intently or cry, I'd go to her.

Around the same time I noticed something else: perhaps Leah was showing tired signs after all. About forty minutes after getting up for the day, she would have a lull in energy and move a bit slower. One morning, I tried putting her down for a nap instead of heading out to the mom-and-baby group; she fell asleep right away on her own and slept for two hours—her longest nap in four months. From then on, she began her first nap about an hour after waking up, and slept for one to two and a half hours. But she still resisted afternoon naps. I began leaving her in her crib for an hour whether she slept or not, going in to reassure her if she cried. During her naps, she often woke after about forty minutes and called out with an "I-am-still-tired" cry; when I let her settle back into sleep, she napped for another hour or so and woke up calm and happy.

Shifting her naps led to a much earlier bedtime of 7 p.m. With this early bedtime, Leah still went to sleep on her own after chatting for a bit. She was back to two night wakings.

At nine and a half months, Leah was still waking up twice, but she now stayed awake for quite a while. I held her, but she usually wanted to either comfort-nurse or play rather than sleep. One night Jason went in with a bottle, but she barely fed and wanted to play instead. Perhaps she was no longer hungry at night? We decided that Jason would try going in and holding her instead of feeding. Leah woke twice that night, four times the following night, and made a few sleepy noises the night after that. And then she began sleeping soundly 7 p.m. to 7 a.m.

Fast forward beyond the first year: Leah transitioned to one nap a day at nineteen months and continued napping regularly until she was four and a half yeas old. I now think that my super alert baby who was "never tired" had, in fact, higher-than-average sleep needs, and quickly became overtired. Her sleep rhythm fell into place when I realized that she needed more sleep—and gave her opportunities to become better rested.

Keeping you close: Emily and Jack

When Emily was pregnant with Jack, she knew one thing for sure: she would keep him close, day and night. Jack was her third— and likely her last—baby.

Jack arrived in the middle of the night in a fast and intense home birth as soon as Emily's pregnancy reached full term. That night, he slept in his parents' bed, as he would for many nights after that. Emily had prepared the space for bed-sharing ahead of time: a large firm mattress on the floor, with no pillows. She lay on her side, facing Jack, with her knees bent, creating a nest. She wore a long-sleeved pyjama top and didn't pull a blanket above her waist.

In the early weeks, Emily went to bed with Jack, nursing him to sleep and whenever he stirred at night. Jack seemed sensitive to loud noises, bright lights, and sudden changes in his surroundings; he communicated his discontent loudly and clearly. During the day Emily carried him in a wrap most of the time. Jack was calm that way and nursed when he wanted.

When Jack was eight weeks old, Emily noticed that his last nap of the day—which usually began just after dinner—was really his bedtime, as he would often fall back asleep for the night right upon waking from this nap. She began giving Jack a bath around 7 p.m., nursing him to sleep, and placing him in a bassinet by her bed. She would nurse him again before she went to bed herself and keep him in bed with her for the rest of the night. Jack nursed frequently, but Emily didn't keep track of how often.

By six months, Jack had a consistent routine. On weekdays, he woke up for the day just after 7 a.m. and accompanied Emily and his older brothers on a walk to school; he napped in the wrap on the way back for half an hour. On weekends, Jack usually took a morning nap in the crib, and then napped for a couple of hours in the afternoon in bed with Emily as she read or slept.

Soon Emily noticed that on weekdays Jack looked tired, was irritable most of the afternoon and early evening, and took longer to drift off to sleep at night. Emily realized that the short nap he was having on weekday mornings was likely not enough to give him the rest he needed and that he was letting her know in the only way he could. She looked at the family's daily routine, gave it some thought, and changed things around. Her partner started taking the children to school on Mondays and a neighbour walked with them on Tuesdays and Fridays. On those days Jack took longer morning naps at home; on the remaining two weekdays he still napped in a wrap during the school walk, but Emily shifted his bedtime to an earlier hour to compensate for the shorter nap.

Jack is now three years old. He still bed-shares with his parents, but has recently asked if he can have a sleepover in his brothers' room. "As long as we can keep the early bedtime for all the kids... maybe he's ready," Emily said to her partner. "And are you ready?" he asked. No... she's not ready yet, but she'll listen to Jack and let him decide when he's ready: after all, he has always let her know.

The gift of time: Tessa's sleep story

I hadn't envisioned a postpartum babymoon when preparing for my second daughter's arrival, but I got one. A difficult birth left me homebound and unable to lift anything heavier than my baby for a month. It ended up being a physically challenging yet special time, as all I needed to do was heal and get to know Tessa. Jason, family, and close friends generously took care of the rest.

By then I knew a lot about baby sleep; I also had an open mind and time to think, watch, and wonder. I wanted to eventually arrive at a point where Tessa slept on her own, but where both she and I knew that if she needed me, she could call and I'd be there for her. I wanted her to be in tune with her body and to see sleep as safe and pleasant. To get there, my goals were to help her stay well-rested and to gently guide her toward independent sleep.

Tessa came into the world strong, calm, and gentle. In the early weeks, she would sleep for a long stretch of two to four hours during the day, nurse for an hour, and go back to sleep. She was a big baby and gained weight well, so our doctor did not suggest waking her for feedings. At night, she slept in short stretches and stayed awake and alert for an hour and a half in between. To support a gradual shift from the "day-night confusion" to more night sleep, I left the curtains open during the day and kept the room dark and quiet at night. In those early weeks, I accepted the ultimate gift of time with my new baby: I slept next to her when she slept in her in-bed bassinet; I watched her quietly; and I slowly got to discover Tessa, myself and Jason as parents of two, and Leah as big sister.

By five weeks, Tessa had consolidated most of her sleep into nighttime. She was going to bed at around 11 p.m. after a simple but consistent bedtime routine of a warm bath and a long feed, would wake up around 3:30 a.m. and again at 6 a.m., and then get up for the day around 9 a.m. During the day she would alternate between forty-minute naps and wakeful periods of about an hour and twenty minutes, sometimes less. Most of the time she'd fall asleep nursing, but when she didn't, I would put her in her bassinet and lie beside her, gently stroking her forehead; sometimes she'd drift off to sleep on her own and sometimes she wouldn't. Holding her upright a certain way against my body for ten minutes after a feeding helped her burp and made her more comfortable before bed.

By seven weeks, Tessa was going to bed at 9 p.m., waking up twice to feed, and getting up for the day at 8 a.m. She stopped falling asleep while nursing at bedtime, but would drift off with a pacifier while I stayed near and held my hand on her forehead. I found it helped to do the last step of our bedtime routine with lights off; otherwise the change startled her. I also found that Tessa needed her diaper changed several times during the night, but she stayed more settled and relaxed if I changed her after she fed for a while. Following the diaper change she would feed some more and drift off to sleep.

At two and a half months, Tessa was going to bed just after 7 p.m., waking to nurse once or twice, and getting up at 6:30 a.m. Her awake windows between naps were still about an hour and twenty minutes long, and her naps were still short. She took most of her naps in the crib now, but I carried her in a wrap for her late afternoon nap as we went for a walk in our neighbourhood.

By three and a half months Tessa's first morning nap lengthened to over an hour on most days. She was now taking three naps a day and falling asleep on her own as I stayed in a chair beside her. She no longer used a pacifier, but began sucking her fingers. She woke to nurse only once most nights.

At four and a half months, however, Tessa began waking frequently at night and staying awake for a while, often an hour or more. Sometimes she re-settled on her own; when she called me, I nursed her. No one was getting much sleep around that time; even when Tessa did not call out we could still hear her rustling, babbling, and rolling from side to side. I knew that I could quickly nurse or hold her back to sleep, but that would not give her a chance to practise settling on her own. I found it challenging to let Tessa stay awake like that and worried that she was getting overtired. She took two naps during the day, each one and a half to two hours long; when she seemed tired or cranky in the late afternoon we either fit in another nap or moved her bedtime to 6 p.m.

At six months, Tessa began sleeping on her tummy. She still woke a lot at night. She was now sleeping in her own room and our bedtime routine was longer: bath, massage, a book, a song, and a feeding. She self-settled for some wakings and I nursed her when she called. But now if she asked to nurse less than two hours after the last feeding, Jason would tell her it was time to rest and stayed with her if she got upset.

When Tessa was seven months old, we went on a two-week-long trip. We kept her routine as similar to our home routine as possible and helped her gradually adjust to the new time zone. I expected her sleep to become disorganized during the trip, but she woke only once or twice per night. A couple of weeks after we returned home Tessa began sleeping from 6:30 p.m. to 6:30 a.m., with naps at 9 a.m. and 2 p.m.

Fast forward beyond the first year: Tessa transitioned to one nap a day at sixteen months and napped every day until she turned five. Now at age 6, she goes to bed at around 7:30 p.m. and enjoys her usual bedtime routine, which is still one of my favourite parts of the day.

When you want to make a change

There are many definitions of infant sleep problems, but I won't get into describing them because I don't think generic "sleep problems" exist. There are simply arrangements and approaches that do not work—or no longer work—for your baby or for you.

When that happens, it is absolutely okay to change course, as long as your new vision is safe, respectful, and consistent.

You are probably looking into making changes because you're not getting enough sleep, your baby's not getting enough sleep, or both. Let's take a look at what might be happening and what you can do.

You need more sleep

Let's start with a case where your baby is sleeping well, but *you* are not getting enough sleep (probably a rare case, I know). Needing and wanting more sleep yourself is not at all selfish: sleep is crucial for your physical and mental health. And changing your own sleep setting may help a great deal.

If you're having trouble falling asleep or are sleeping restlessly because of worries and anxiety—which is known as postpartum insomnia—consider changing where you sleep. If your baby is older and you room-share, it might help you to sleep in another room so you don't wake up each time baby shifts position. Or, if your baby sleeps separately from you, you may find that room-sharing brings you peace of mind and allows you to sleep better. Also, don't forget the usual sleep advice you would have turned to pre-baby: watch your caffeine intake, don't use screens before bed, and consider meditation and relaxation techniques.

If you're feeling tired because of fragmented sleep (for example, because of your baby feeding frequently at night), look for ways to get more sleep and rest. Nap when your baby naps, if you can. Ask your partner or a family member to take over a feeding or two. Remember, really sleepless nights will pass soon. If you're experiencing extreme fatigue, do ask for help (and don't forget to look into causes other than sleep, such as low iron or thyroid issues).

Your baby needs more sleep (and I bet so do you)

Do you feel your baby is not getting enough rest? Let's go back and look at the building blocks of sound sleep on page 49.

First, ask yourself whether your **vision** and **expectations** of your baby's sleep are developmentally appropriate. Young babies have very fragmented sleep, and older babies may still need to feed several times at night.

Next, think about your baby's **sleeping space**. Is there anything you can do to make the space more comfortable (such as making it darker, cooler, or quieter)? Can you give your baby more regular opportunities to nap in his usual sleeping space at home?

Next, look at your bedtime and middle-of-the-night routines from a standpoint of **sleep associations**. Consider what happens, where and how it happens, and who is present. Is there anything you can do to bring in more consistency, create familiar and comforting patterns, and help your baby recognize these patterns?

Finally, take a really good look at your baby's **daily rhythm**. For at least five days, keep a sleep diary. Look at your baby's morning wake-up time, naps, bedtime, and awake times in between. Compare them with those described in the stage-by-stage guide on pages 64–83. Could your baby's sleep timing use some adjustment? Consider shifting bedtime to an earlier hour. Remember, day and night sleep are interrelated: both night and day sleep tend to improve when the day-sleep rhythm is adjusted,[133] so take a really good look at your baby's naps. For example, you may want to help him start his first nap earlier or re-establish a second nap.

Make a plan: think through your new sleep vision. Check your vision for consistency, from both your own and your baby's perspective. Write down all the changes you're going to introduce under "sleeping space," "sleep associations," and "sleep rhythm." Discuss these changes with your partner and any other caregivers in your baby's life.

Now you're ready to **introduce the changes**. Begin by making all the changes you wrote down under "sleeping space" and "daily rhythm." Why start with those? Because adjusting your baby's sleeping space and timing will be straightforward, won't be upsetting for your baby, and may be all you need to do to get to (or back to) sound sleep. For example, you may want to make the room darker and quieter, give baby more regular opportunities for napping at home, encourage her to take her first nap within an hour and a half after waking, and move her bedtime earlier. Once you introduce these changes, be consistent and observe carefully. Wait at least a week to see if your baby's sleep improves. Continue your sleep diary so you can track the changes.

If you're not seeing improvement, introduce the changes you wrote down under "sleep associations." Your baby will need time to adjust and get to know the new patterns. He may feel upset by the changes and protest, especially if where he sleeps or how he goes to sleep is now different. No matter how small the changes, tell your baby about them. "Tonight we will start your bath right after we come back from the walk, instead of playing in the den"; "Daddy and I have moved your crib into your room. Let's go and take a look. Today you'll be in your crib for your afternoon nap."

You probably noticed I haven't yet used the term "sleep training." Well, this is where it *may* come in. Many approaches have been developed, ranging from the slow and gentle "no cry" solutions to detached and efficient "extinction" or "cry it out" without the caregiver. In my mind, all of them have the same goal—arriving at a point where baby has sustainable sleep associations—but they propose very different paths to getting there. In other words, the approaches differ in *how* the baby gets to a point of self-settling during wakings when he has no need greater than sleep. Whether and how much crying will be involved depends on the approach you choose and on your baby's temperament.

Choose the approach you feel most comfortable with. I cannot tell you which one to use, but here are some questions to guide you:

- How do you feel about crying?
- Can you tell the difference between an expression of protest (a want) and distress (a need)? Is your baby old enough and communicating enough for you to reliably tell these apart?
- It is not the practice in crying, but the practice in going to sleep under new conditions, that will bring sound sleep to your baby. Letting a baby cry first and then switching to rocking her to sleep will be hard on both of you and won't get you any closer to sound sleep. Will you be able to consistently use the approach you're choosing? Does it feel right to you?

Below I list four resources for further reading that focus on specific techniques and the logic behind them. That being said, you don't have to use any particular formula. It's okay to combine different ideas to come up with your own approach, as long as it's safe, respectful, and consistent.

Techniques for Sleep Problem Solving: Suggested Reading

- *Healthy Sleep Habits, Happy Child: A step-by-step program for a good night's sleep,* 4th ed., by Marc Weissbluth (2015) Dr. Weissbluth is a pediatrician and a sleep researcher who coined the term "sleep training" and authored a number of landmark studies establishing the importance of sleep schedule for children. In this sourcebook he describes multiple sleep-training methods including "extinction" ("cry it out").

- *The Happy Sleeper: A science-backed guide to helping your baby get a good night's sleep—newborn to school age,* by Heather Turgeon and Julie Wright (2014) The focus of this book is on helping babies develop self-soothing skills. The authors describe how to set healthy sleep habits from the start and suggest solutions to sleep problems. The main solution (the "Sleep Wave") involves letting baby fall asleep on her own with regular checks by the parent. Includes a section for bed-sharing families.
- *The Sleep Book for Tired Parents: Help for solving children's sleep problems,* by Rebecca Huntley (1991) This book lays out four approaches to solving sleep problems, without advocating for any particular one: the Family Bed, Cry It Out, Small Steps, and Living with It. It is written in a workbook format and includes an exercise to help parents determine which approach is likely to work best for them.
- *The No-Cry Sleep Solution,* by Elizabeth Pantley (2002) The focus of this book is on changing sleep habits and daily routines. The changes are introduced slowly, with more work and with little to no crying. Advice is very relevant for bed-sharing families, but also helpful to families whose babies sleep solo.

Once you choose your approach, be very consistent and give it time to work. It may take from a few days to several months. But no matter the methods, from very gentle to more direct, you *will* see results as long as you are truly consistent.

This section would not be complete without one more thought. There is nothing wrong with intentionally choosing to *not* make a change. There may be special circumstances involved (for example, an illness or a medical condition) or you may simply want to wait it out. Recognize that you have intentionally chosen to not change things for now—and that's okay. Be mindful of how rested your baby is, how rested your family is, and how you're feeling. Re-examine your decision when you feel the need to.

Questions you may have

Q **Building the sleep foundation seems like a lot of work. Is it really necessary? And when will I get my "me time" back?**

A Staying close to home, observing, and carefully adjusting the daily rhythm does take commitment, time, and patience. It really does. But this approach will help your baby stay well-rested, which will support the development of his sleep structure to benefit him for life. Careful observation will also help you get to know your baby; try to think of it not as "work," but as a unique and special time. Once baby's bedtime shifts to the early evening (between 6 and 8 p.m.; usually by three months), you will be able to reclaim some grown-up time in the evenings; when your baby begins taking naps at consistent times, usually by eight months, you'll also be able to enjoy more predictable breaks during the day.

Q **How can I tell whether my baby is well-rested?**

A When your baby is young, it might be hard to tell how rested she is; give her consistent and plentiful opportunities for rest and trust your intuition. Once your baby is six months or older, you can gauge how rested she is by answering the following questions. Does your baby generally have a predictable sleep pattern? Does she usually wake up on her own, looking content, in the morning and after naps? If you answered yes to both questions, your baby is likely well-rested.

Q I've heard that if I feed my baby to sleep, he won't sleep well. Is it better to not include feeding in my baby's sleep routine?

A I think feeding is a very intuitive, natural element of a sleep routine. In the early weeks, your baby will likely drift off to sleep during or after a feeding. As she gets older, a well-rested baby is likely to stop falling asleep while feeding. This could be a natural start to practising self-settling if you plan to have your baby sleep solo. If your baby sleeps with you and you're breastfeeding, you could comfort-nurse until she's asleep or help her drift off to sleep by cuddling, stroking her head, or using another soothing approach that works for you and your baby (and, importantly, is sustainable for you to repeat in the middle of the night).

Q What about the "dream feed"?

A Many popular baby sleep resources recommend a "dream feed": gently rousing and feeding the baby around the time you go to bed yourself, without fully waking him. The idea is that this feeding will fill your baby's tummy and buy you a longer stretch of uninterrupted sleep. But remember that babies tend to sleep very deeply early in the night. If you try to feed your baby then, he may not be awake enough to take a full feeding. Or, he may wake up fully and have trouble going back to sleep as his sleep rhythms get out of sync. It is also difficult to decide when to stop dream feeding because you cannot rely on your baby's cues as you would have otherwise.

Q I want my baby to sleep separately from me, but we don't have a lot of space. When can I move her to sleep with an older sibling?

A At the time I write this, the American Academy of Pediatrics recommends that babies sleep in their parents' room until they are twelve months old.[111] After that they can sleep in their own room or room-share, but not bed-share, with siblings.[148] Before making the move, think about the best way to maintain familiar routines and appropriate bedtimes for all the children. Talk about the changes with all of them, including the baby, ahead of time.

Q I'm going back to work. How can I best support my baby's sleep while I'm away from him?

A If a nanny or a family member will be caring for your baby, talk to them about your approaches and beliefs. Ask them to read this book or parts of it. Write down your baby's routines and usual nap times. The caregiver does not have to follow your sleep routines exactly, but asking them to bring in some elements of your usual routine will help your baby settle for sleep more easily.

If your baby is going to attend a daycare centre, discuss the centre's sleep approaches and share yours ahead of time. Send in a familiar blanket or a sleep-safe cuddle toy if your baby has one. Write a one-page note describing your baby's routines, usual nap times, and what helps your baby settle for sleep. Talk with your baby's primary caregiver and touch base with them at the end of each day to see, among other things, how much rest your baby got that day. Don't lose the early bedtime; this is easier said than done, I know, but even more important now.

Q **When will my baby sleep through the night?**

A As you now know, there's no straight answer to this question. The age at which a baby no longer needs night feeds differs from baby to baby. Not to mention the fact that what you and I consider sleeping through the night might be two completely different things. By creating an environment that supports sleep development, you are helping your baby begin sleeping *as soundly as he can as early as he is ready.*

Watch and Wonder

If you can't figure out your baby's tired signs, keep watching: tomorrow will bring new opportunities. Remember that you're not doing anything wrong.

At bedtime, create a feeling of safety and warmth around your baby. Start a tradition of recapping the day and talking about tomorrow for a sense of flow. It may seem too early to be doing this, but it will be good for both of you.

Watch your baby sleep. Think about how remarkable it is that everyone you know was once a baby this small.

Take pictures of your baby's sleeping space at different stages. Take pictures of your baby sleeping. Videotape your bedtime routine by putting a camera in auto mode.

Think about whether your sleep arrangement is still working for you, your baby, and the rest of the family. If it isn't, will you choose to make adjustments or changes? Why or why not?

Trust that you will find sound sleep.

On an extra-long-nap day or when your partner or a family member is looking after your baby, do what makes you feel nourished and cared for. That could mean traditional self-care activities like a nap, shower, or a cup of tea with a friend to nourish your body or soul. Or it might mean taking care of a chore or task you've been waiting to do, in order to free up your mind. Either way, don't feel guilty or as if you should have done something else.

On an extra-short-nap day, take your baby for a long walk in the stroller or baby carrier. He may or may not nap, but you both will get fresh air.

Remember that you cannot make your baby sleep. You are responsible for *letting* her sleep, but not for *making* her sleep.

The next chapter will explore eating and feeding—and what you can do to create a feeding environment that's as healthy and supportive as possible.

CHAPTER 3
FEEDING

Open wide, here comes the airplane

Babies have very high nutritional needs: they are growing and developing faster than they ever will. Babyhood also sets the foundation for future eating. Eating patterns and food preferences are known to take shape early in life and continue into adulthood.[149]

Feeding provides us with one of the best opportunities to get to know our babies and to enjoy each other's company. It can feel meaningful and deeply satisfying, but it can also become a source of worry or frustration.

In developed countries in the twenty-first century, children's eating habits form under conditions of unprecedented abundance:[150] most families with adequate resources have access to a wide variety of foods from around the world, year-round. With so many options and opinions about what is healthy and what is not, it can be difficult to decide what to feed your baby and how to do it. And it can be even more difficult to feel confident and supported in your choices. Let's take a look at what science can tell us about first foods, eating skills development, and feeding dynamics during baby's first year.

PART I
THE SCIENCE OF EATING AND FEEDING

Milk

You have probably come across the debate of whether "breast is best." The short answer from science is this: yes, breastmilk is the optimal food for babies. Although breastmilk and formula milk have similar nutritional value, breastmilk also contains bioactive components that protect babies against infection, support immune system development, and help nutrient absorption.[151] These are very important and unique benefits. Breastfed babies tend to have several other advantages later in life such as increased intelligence and well-being, but it is not certain whether these result from breastmilk itself or from other aspects of the overall home environment. Boxes that follow have the details.

In addition to health benefits, breastmilk is always clean, free, and better for our planet: there are no manufacturing costs and no need for packaging or disposal, apart from a few supplies breastfeeding families may choose to purchase.

> **Unique Benefits of Breastmilk**
>
> **Breastmilk provides immune support**: The child's immune system does not reach full strength until adolescence, and even then it continues to evolve.[152] Breastmilk helps babies avoid and fight off illness in several ways. First, through mother's immune response,

antibodies develop in breastmilk to target pathogens *in baby's immediate surroundings*. Breastmilk is, quite literally, an ounce of prevention delivered at just the right time to keep baby healthy! Second, milk invigorates the baby's own immune response.[152] Milk has inactive enzymes that get activated in baby's digestive tract to further aid the immune system.[153] Such immune support is unique to breastmilk and is not offered by formula. Its benefits can be seen in several ways, for example:

- Premature babies fed breastmilk have significantly lower incidence of necrotizing enterocolitis (a devastating intestinal infection that often affects preemies), especially when fed their own mother's milk or donor milk from another mother who delivered early: such milk has extra protein and bioactive components to support the baby's immune system.[154, 155]
- Breastfed babies produce more antibodies in response to immunizations,[156] which shows that they have stronger immune systems.
- Children who were breastfed for longer periods of time have better lung growth.[157]

Breastmilk helps microbiome development: In the last few years, studies have begun showing the effects of breastmilk on the microorganisms in a baby's digestive system. Communities of these microorganisms are called the microbiota, or the gut flora, and their composition is called the microbiome. The microbiome is essential for immune and metabolic health[153, 158] and has even been considered a separate organ from a physiological standpoint.[159] In the womb, babies are believed to have no microorganisms at all,[160] but the microbiome begins to assemble immediately after birth. Many factors affect microbiome development, but the main ones are how baby was born (vaginally or through a C-section), whether antibiotics were administered, and the type of milk—breastmilk or formula—baby receives.[158, 161] Breastmilk contains probiotics (elements of the mother's microbiome) and prebiotics (sugar polymers that feed beneficial microbiota).[153] The synergy of these pro- and prebiotics supports beneficial bifidobacteria in a baby's digestive system and provides breastfed babies with a more stable and uniform microbiome compared to formula-fed babies.[158] The milk-microbiome connection may explain why those who were breastfed are less likely to develop immune-mediated health conditions later in life.[161]

Breastmilk acts as a flavour bridge: When solid foods are first introduced, breastfed babies are often more enthusiastic about eating than formula-fed babies. There is a neat mechanism behind this. Many flavours from the mother's diet appear in her breastmilk, and so breastfed babies are already used to experiencing a wide variety of tastes.[162,163] In contrast, formula offers the same consistent flavour day after day. That being said, formula-fed babies can and do learn to enjoy a variety of foods as well, they might just need a little extra time and patience.

These are scientifically proven benefits of breastmilk.

Benefits Associated with Breastfeeding
(which may or may not be caused by the breastmilk itself)

Increased intelligence: Many studies have shown that babies fed breastmilk score higher on intelligence tests later in life, as older children[164-168] and as adults.[151] Neurophysiological studies offer explanations: children who were breastfed generally have larger brains and more grey and white brain matter.[166,168] However, it's difficult to determine if breastmilk alone or the overall parenting style and home environment are responsible for these benefits.[169] In other words, are other social and family characteristics that breastfeeding is typically associated with causing most or all of the difference? Well-designed studies that found associations between breastmilk and increased intelligence did statistically adjust for some parent and family characteristics, such as income and education. However, unsurprisingly, neither income nor education is a perfect measure of the parents' intelligence.[170] Studying siblings—where parents' intelligence is the same but one sibling was fed breastmilk and the other formula— is one way to test whether parental intelligence plays a part. Such studies showed only a small IQ advantage for breastfed siblings over those who were formula-fed.[170-172] Another way is to directly measure, and statistically adjust for, the mothers' IQ—and when this was done, breastfeeding advantage was again very small.[170]

Better mental health and well-being: Several studies have shown that babies who were breastfed, especially for six months or longer, had better mental health as older children, adolescents, and adults (they were less likely to develop anxiety, attention problems, or delinquent and aggressive behaviour).[173,174] Similar to the research on intelligence, these studies accounted for a number of other factors such as parents' age, education, and income, family structure, and stressful childhood events. However, other unmeasured characteristics of babies' environment might have contributed to the differences.

So, does breastfeeding make babies smarter and happier? Science will never be able to answer these questions with full certainty: it is not possible to raise the same baby twice and note the differences, and it's not ethical to randomly assign babies to "breastmilk" and "formula" groups and look at the outcomes. Future studies may add more weight to either hypothesis, but no scientific measurements and adjustments will ever fully capture the complexity of what makes someone "smart" and "happy"—big concepts that mean different things to different people anyway.

Breastfeeding

If you** choose to breastfeed, you will likely be able to: most women can.[175] Breastfeeding may come easily or you may experience challenges in the first few days or weeks.

** Unlike most parts of this book, here "you" refers to the breastfeeding mother, but if you are her partner or family member, please keep reading. This section will help you understand and support her on her breastfeeding journey.

Common breastfeeding challenges

Most women encounter at least some difficulties in the early days of breastfeeding,[176] but the majority of them can be resolved with knowledge and support.

After their birth, babies feed on colostrum, the pre-milk rich in immune-supporting components. Milk usually comes in twenty-four to 102 hours after birth—a fairly wide range—but for most women it happens on day three.[177]

It is very common for breastfeeding mothers to experience nipple soreness and discomfort.[178,179] This discomfort usually goes away after a few days. Persistent discomfort or pain usually indicates that the baby does not have a deep enough latch: she is not getting enough breast tissue into her mouth.

Improper latch is one of the most common breastfeeding challenges.[178,180] Sometimes it's caused by the baby's or mother's position during breastfeeding and requires only a small adjustment. Other times it's caused by structural issues such as a mother's inverted nipples or baby's tongue or lip ties.[178] A tongue tie means that the baby's frenulum—the membrane under his tongue—is unusually thick, tight, or short, restricting the tongue's movement. Similarly, an upper lip tie can restrict upper lip movement. Tongue ties are reported in 3 to 11 percent of babies, but the true percentage may be higher because not all cases are documented. Most babies with tongue or lip ties cannot create a vacuum as they latch onto the breast; some cannot latch at all, while others can but are less efficient at extracting milk because of decreased tongue mobility. Their mothers often experience nipple pain and damage, breast pain, and mastitis.[181] Frenotomy, a small surgical procedure in which the frenulum is cut, makes breastfeeding more comfortable, improves milk production, and leads to more efficient feedings.[181-183] For babies with tongue ties, frenotomy has been proven safe and much more effective in resolving improper latch than improving the feeding position or adjusting feeding frequency.[184]

Although most lactation consultants agree that tongue ties cause breastfeeding difficulties, not all pediatricians do, and many medical guidelines don't specify whether tongue ties need to be treated; because of this, families often receive conflicting advice on whether their baby has a tongue or lip tie and whether a frenotomy is recommended.[181]

Responsive breastfeeding

In the past, mothers were advised to breastfeed on a schedule, but we now know that babies should be fed on demand. I prefer the term *responsive breastfeeding*: following baby's cues for when and how much to feed. (Baby's only way of *demanding* to be fed, crying, is a *late* hunger cue; we'll talk about how to tell when your baby is hungry in Part II of this chapter.)

Why is it important to breastfeed responsively? Babies are able to feed according to appetite from birth,[177] consume exactly what they need,[185] and, by doing so, establish and maintain their mother's milk supply.[186] Breastfeeding responsively allows babies to eat when they're hungry and stop when they're full, helping them retain their natural ability to feed according to their appetite.[187, 188]

Breastfeeding Myths

Myth #1: *Nursing mothers should follow a certain diet.* What the mother eats does not significantly affect her milk composition or production, so generally there is no need to avoid any food groups (unless advised to by a health care practitioner). A balanced diet rich in vitamins and minerals is best for the mother's health and well-being; some components, including brain-building omega-3 fatty acids, do transfer to the baby through breastmilk.[189]

Myth #2: *Babies who feed frequently do not get enough high-fat milk.* Some babies tend to take frequent small feeds while other babies like to space larger feeds farther apart.[186] Mothers of frequent feeders are often concerned that their babies are not getting enough of the high-fat hindmilk that comes later in a feed. While it is true that hindmilk is *generally* higher in fat, the fat content also adapts to the frequency of feedings, so the total amount of fat babies get over the course of the day is about the same regardless of whether they feed frequently or not.[177]

Myth #3: *Pacifiers ruin breastfeeding.* For mothers who are highly motivated to breastfeed, the recommendation to offer or not offer a pacifier does not appear to affect the prevalence or duration of breastfeeding.[190] Overall, research suggests that pacifier use is a matter of preference rather than a health decision; it is best to introduce it after breastfeeding is established, offer it for sleep during the first year,[191] and not use it for prolonged periods beyond baby's first birthday.[192]

Myth #4: *Breast fullness is a good indicator of milk production.* Milk production and the volume of milk babies drink per day becomes fully established by about one month and remains fairly constant until six months.[186] After that, breast tissue decreases, but milk production can still be high. Lesser breast fullness does not necessarily equal less milk.[177,178]

Breastmilk is the best choice for every baby, but may not be a possibility or the right choice for every family. We are fortunate to have the option of safe, nutritionally adequate, and widely available formula milk.

Formula feeding

As the science on infant development and nutrition progresses, formula milk is constantly being improved to better meet babies' needs. For example, omega-3 fatty acids, especially docosahexaenoic acid (DHA), are important for brain maturation and for vision.[193] In the 1980s studies began to show that babies who were fed formula—which at the time contained no DHA—had lower levels of DHA and poorer vision acuity compared to breastfed babies.[189] Formula now contains DHA and other omega-3 fatty acids.[194]

Very recently, formulas enriched with certain oligosaccharides (prebiotics) have been developed. Babies fed these formulas have more bifidobacteria in their digestive systems and their microbiomes are more similar, although not identical, to microbiomes of breastfed babies.[161, 195] At the time I write this in 2020, not all formula contains prebiotics.

Solid food

When babies approach the middle of their first year, complementary foods commonly known as "solid foods" or "table foods" are gradually introduced alongside breastmilk or formula.

When to start

You might have heard that "Food before one is just for fun." This adage is used with good intentions—to promote longer breastfeeding and to reassure parents—but it is not entirely true.

The advice on when to introduce solid foods varies across countries, but it generally falls somewhere between four and six months. At the time I write this, the World Health Organization recommends that "infants start receiving complementary foods at six months of age in addition to breast milk." This is because from about six months on, breastmilk is no longer enough as the only source of some of the essential nutrients such as iron. Starting at around six months, babies are exceedingly at risk of iron deficiency: by then they've depleted the iron stores they had at birth and their diets tend to be low in iron, but their needs are high due to rapid growth.[196] It is partly for this reason that the period from six to twelve months is recognized as one of the most nutritionally vulnerable times in childhood.

That being said, it is also important to be aware of, and appreciate, the individual differences between babies: some are ready for solid foods earlier and others need extra time. From a gross motor and oral motor development perspective, the two main signs of readiness are the ability to sit upright and the disappearance of the tongue-thrust reflex.[197] It's also important to consider babies' interest in table foods and their ability to communicate hunger and satiety. Healthy, full-term babies develop motor skills and mealtime communication skills at different times. Here are the common milestones.[197, 198]

Ability	Commonly emerges around	Normal range
Opens mouth when hungry	4.5 months	Birth to 9 months
Sits upright on caregiver's lap	5.5 months	3 to 10 months
Closes mouth to reject food	6 months	1 to 11 months
Brings upper lip down on spoon to remove food	7.5 months	4 to 16 months
Eats foods with small lumps without gagging	8.5 months	5 to 15 months
Eats finger foods	8.5 months	6 to 12 months
Chews foods, keeps most in mouth	9 months	6 to 14 months

Notice how wide the ranges are for each milestone. One healthy six-month-old baby may demonstrate all of these abilities, while another may not yet show any of them, yet both babies would be within the normal ranges of development.

Our role in feeding

Appetite and responsive feeding

Remarkably, babies can regulate how much they eat depending on a food's nutritional density. Back in the 1920s, pioneering research[199, 200] showed that babies and children can thrive on self-selected diets when allowed to eat according to their appetites. The box below describes this unique work. In a more recent study, four- to six-month-old babies who were exclusively breastfed showed the same energy intake and growth as babies who were fed breastmilk and solid food, suggesting that all babies self-regulated how much they ate.[201]

All On Their Own

In the 1920s and 1930s, Dr. Clara Davis and her team carried out unusual research[199, 200] that changed the thinking on children's eating. The scientists followed fifteen babies from four months to six years old. Every day at every meal the children were offered the same selection of thirty-four foods, each served in a separate little dish, and then allowed to eat whatever and how much they wanted, with no adult influence. The foods came from both plant and animal sources, provided all the necessary nutrients, were available fresh year-round, and required only very simple preparation.

The results? Every child's diet was different from every other child's diet, but none showed the cereal and milk dominance with small amounts of fruit, eggs, and meat that was commonly thought to be proper for babies and children at the time. Meals often included strange-from-the-adult-perspective combinations (a breakfast of orange juice and liver, anyone?). All foods except lettuce were tried by all children, especially in the early weeks, but distinct tastes formed over time. As children grew, they changed how much protein they consumed as their body weight changed, consistent with the change in energy requirements that comes with growth and increased activity. Children who took no or very little cow's milk for considerable periods of time still developed strong bones. All children grew healthy and strong, even those who had rickets at the beginning of the study.

Scientists believe that the "trick" in this study was the food list: successful eating of self-selected diets by appetite was possible because only natural, healthy foods were offered. If overly sweet or salty fried foods had been included in their day-to-day diet, children would have likely developed a preference for these energy-dense but nutrient-poor choices,[149] and the outcomes would have been different.

Babies are born capable of eating well. But to retain these capabilities and to continue tuning in to their sensations as they grow, they need supportive feeding environments.

Control or pressure during feeding reduces a child's ability to self-regulate.[149] In one study, when mothers were responsive in their feeding, babies self-corrected their growth trajectories: those who gained weight slowly in the early months began growing faster between six and twelve months. But when mothers were controlling—for example, forcing, repositioning, or distracting their babies in an effort to make them eat more—the opposite pattern was observed: smaller babies grew even slower. This shows that controlling is, in fact, counterproductive.[202] Controlling overrides babies' internal hunger and satiety clues.[203]

To help families with feeding, Ellyn Satter developed the Division of Responsibility concept,[204] also known as responsive feeding:[205]

- Parents are responsible for the When, What, and Where of feeding; they set a nurturing feeding environment and predictably provide nutritious foods.
- Children are responsible for the How Much and Whether of eating; they decide how much of each food to eat and whether to eat it at all.

Children fed responsively tend to eat better nutritionally and are more likely to be of healthy weight.[206]

Purees and baby-led weaning

Traditionally, babies begin eating smooth purees fed by a spoon, progress to lumpy textures, and eventually begin eating small pieces of food. Baby-led weaning (or BLW for short) is a different approach that has recently become quite popular: instead of being spoon-fed by adults, babies feed themselves hand-held food from the very beginning. One of the main benefits of this approach is that baby chooses and controls how much and how fast she eats.[206] There have been several studies on this subject so far. They suggest the following:

- BLW is feasible for many, but not all six-month-olds from a motor development perspective.[207]
- BLW gives babies more control over their eating. In addition, during BLW babies tend to gum or munch on their food, which helps with digestion. Young babies have most of the enzymes needed to digest starches in their saliva (unlike adults and older children who produce these enzymes in the pancreas).[4]
- One of the main concerns related to BLW is the possibility of choking. To date, studies have found no difference in choking incidents between BLW and spoon-fed babies.[207, 208] Safety considerations important for both styles of feeding include

always closely watching babies during mealtimes and avoiding foods that consist of, or can separate into, firm pieces.

- Another concern related to BLW is the possibility of nutrient deficiencies, and especially iron deficiency. However, when parents are encouraged to offer iron-rich foods at every meal, BLW style results in a diet nutritionally similar to the spoon-fed one[209] and does not appear to increase the risk of iron deficiency.[210]

Accepting new foods: the importance of repeated exposure and variety

Most babies are adventurous and eager when they first begin eating solid foods. The majority of families describe their four- to six-month-olds as "not picky."[211] But as the first year goes by, strong food likes and dislikes may appear, and by twelve months many babies are characterized as picky eaters.[198, 211] What's happening?

What most parents don't realize is that babies may need eight to fifteen tastes of new food, in different meals and in a supportive, no-pressure setting, before they become accustomed to the new flavour.[212, 213] These repeated exposures need to be actual bites, not just seeing or playing with the food. In one study,[213] when offered an initially disliked vegetable over eight subsequent meals, most babies learned to like it as much as their favourite vegetable; nine months later, they still liked it! Yet, most parents offer a food item only a few times, and often just once, before deciding their baby does not like it.[198]

Babies may need eight or more tastes of a new food before they accept (and usually grow to like) the new flavour.

Breastfed babies are more likely to accept a novel food when it's first offered because they have already been exposed, through breastmilk, to a variety of flavour experiences. But after several repeated exposures, formula-fed babies accept novel flavours as well.[162]

Overall, the more experience a baby has with different foods, the greater his willingness to try more will be: babies benefit from a variety in flavours and textures.[214, 215]

Best first foods

Diets vary greatly between cultures and among families, and guidelines on healthy eating tend to change frequently. Because of this, I'm not going to recommend any particular foods here. Instead, I've brought together the knowledge on nutrients that are important for all babies, with some examples to illustrate the main points. When I do mention particular foods, I am referring to whole foods, not the highly processed alternatives or imitation products (for example, "meat" does not include hot dogs).

Nutritious foods: energy and nutrients

As you know, food is a source of energy and nutrients: carbohydrates, fats, proteins, vitamins, minerals, and water. *Energy density* describes how many calories a food has relative to its size or weight. *Nutrient density* is the food's nutrient-to-calories ratio. Given babies' tiny tummies and incredibly fast growth and development, the nutrient density of their food needs to be very high—much higher than what is required for adults.[216]

What foods do you need to avoid during baby's first year? Babies should not be fed honey (of any type) or unpasteurized foods because these carry the risk of botulism.[217] It's best to avoid cow's milk (more on that on page 119). Also, during the first year it is best to avoid foods that are energy-dense but nutrient-poor, such as processed foods high in saturated fat, sugar, or sodium. Examples of highly processed foods include French fries, instant noodles, doughnuts, hot dogs, and sweetened beverages (such as soft drinks). Such foods are "empty calories" that displace energy from nutrient-dense foods and may contain additives that are harmful if consumed in large amounts.

What are the best foods to offer? As long as breastmilk and/or formula continues to provide essential fats throughout the first year and beyond, the best foods for babies are those that are nutrient-dense, such as:

- Nutrient-dense and energy-dense: meat, fish, eggs, avocado
- Nutrient-dense: vegetables and fruit

Nutrients that are important for babies, but not always abundant in Western diets and environments, are iron and vitamin D.[216, 218] Formula is usually fortified with both. For breastfed and partially breastfed babies, vitamin D is often recommended as a supplement because it is not found in many foods.[219] Iron, however, can come from iron-rich foods and is absorbed best that way.[196]

Iron

From about six months on, babies are exceedingly vulnerable to iron deficiency.[196] Breastmilk is still very important and highly beneficial, but at this age it's no longer sufficient as babies' only source of iron. Iron can come from animal-based foods (heme iron) and plant sources (non-heme iron). Heme iron is more bioavailable: it is absorbed more efficiently (15 to 35 percent of the amount consumed is absorbed) compared to non-heme iron (of which only 3 to 5 percent is absorbed).[220] Examples of foods naturally rich in heme iron are poultry and red (non-processed) meats; these foods also contain beneficial zinc and protein and are low in sodium.[221]

What about baby cereals fortified with iron? Added iron (and sometimes zinc) aside, these cereals are generally made of nutrient- and energy-poor refined grains. The iron within cereals has lower bioavailability:[196,222] it doesn't get absorbed as well as iron from foods like meat. However, fortified cereals can be a source of iron for babies who don't eat enough naturally iron-rich foods.[4,221] Rice cereals, including organic ones, often have concerning levels of arsenic and other heavy metals that can be harmful if consumed regularly.[223] Cereals made from other whole grains, such as oats, quinoa, or amaranth, are generally better choices.

Certain foods help with iron absorption. For example, meats and vitamin C-rich foods improve the absorption of non-heme iron when they're included in the same meal.[224] Other foods, like cow's milk, negatively affect iron status. Cow's milk is low in iron itself and it inhibits the absorption of iron from other foods. Cow's milk was found to cause intestinal blood loss in some (as many as 40 percent) young babies, and although such blood loss was not detected in babies older than twelve months, it is possible that small blood loss still occurs.[225]

Before the agricultural revolution, red meats were likely babies' main source of iron: humans relied on hunting, fishing, and gathering of wild plants, and babies likely consumed a fair amount of pre-chewed, iron-rich meats from wild animals.[216] Meeting babies' needs for iron with modern diets is certainly possible. For example, great sources of heme iron are red meat, poultry, sardines, and egg yolks. Good sources of non-heme iron include white beans, lentils, and spinach.[226] I will share some of my favourite ways to incorporate iron-rich foods into a baby's diet on page 142.

Healthy fats

Healthy fats provide brain-building omega-3 fatty acids, help absorb fat-soluble vitamins (A, D, E, and K), and boost the energy density of foods.[227,228] Fats also make food more sensory appealing and easier to swallow and digest. The best source of fat for babies is breastmilk. Good food sources include egg yolks, especially those from pasture-raised hens,[229] non-processed meat, meat broth, fatty fish, flax oil, olive oil, and avocado.[226]

Vegetables and fruits

Vegetables and fruits are important sources of trace minerals, B vitamins, and fibre. Vitamin C-rich vegetables and fruits increase the absorption of non-heme iron two to six fold. In addition, unless completely pureed, vegetables and fruits have complex textures, which helps develop oral motor skills.[163] Babies who eat abundant fruits, vegetables, and other home-prepared foods during the first year are less likely to develop food allergies by age two.[230]

Studies clearly show the benefits of exploring a variety of vegetables and fruits early on, between five and seven months, both from a nutritional perspective and because babies more readily accept new flavours at this age.[149] Yet a recent survey in the United States showed that, on the day the parents were phoned and asked to complete the survey, one in four six- to twelve-month-olds had had no vegetables at all.[218]

Store-bought or homemade?

A wide selection of commercial baby food jars and pouches, including organic options, is available in stores. These commercial foods are sometimes marketed as superior to home cooked foods, but they are not. Commercial foods are convenient, but less nutritious. A study that looked at a variety of commercial baby foods in the United Kingdom found that they had lower nutrient density compared to similar family foods. For example, a jar of carrot puree was less nutritionally dense than a steamed and pureed whole carrot.[231]

In addition, tastes in store-bought baby foods are often masked by artificial sweetness or the food is quite bland. Such foods do not allow babies to experience—and get accustomed to—richer flavours and textures. Finally, contrary to what many parents think, store-bought baby food is not necessarily subject to more stringent regulation and safety testing than products marketed for adults.[223]

FEEDING: KEY POINTS

- Breastmilk has significant benefits over formula milk: it protects babies against infection, supports immune system development, and helps with nutrient absorption. Breastfeeding challenges are very common, but most can be resolved with knowledge and support.
- Formula milk is a safe alternative that is being continuously improved to meet babies' needs better.
- Solid foods are usually introduced around six months. It's important, however, to consider baby's developmental readiness.
- Babies are born capable of eating well and eating to appetite. To retain these capabilities and continue tuning into their sensations as they grow, they need supportive feeding environments.
- Babies may need eight or more tastes of a new food, in different meals and in a no-pressure setting, before they accept and enjoy the new flavour.
- Given babies' tiny tummies and incredibly fast growth and development, their foods must be nutrient-dense. It is especially important to regularly include iron-rich foods, healthy fats, vegetables, and fruits.

Let's look at how we can best set the stage for healthy and happy eating in our homes.

PART II
A HEALTHY AND HAPPY EATING ENVIRONMENT

Not too long ago we had dinner at a restaurant known for its fresh local cuisine. A couple sitting next to us commented on how great it was to see children enjoying *adult food*. Our daughters were sharing an entrée off the regular menu, not the kids' menu with grilled cheese sandwiches and plain pasta. This friendly comment made me realize that most of us are so used to seeing children eat only a limited number of foods, primarily energy-dense and nutrient-poor ones, that we consider it natural. And our culture supports convenience and rush, offering abundant pre-packaged choices marketed for children.

Offer your baby nutritious foods as much as you can. (I will show you that this doesn't have to be difficult or time-consuming.) Babies cannot advocate for themselves when it comes to eating. When our babies need more sleep, they let us know: lack of sleep quickly affects the whole family, prompting us to look for solutions. But emerging feeding and eating challenges, unless severe, can be hard to spot.

Melissa did not plan on introducing regular screen time so early, but eleven-month-old Evan would simply not eat anything without it. She was able to spoon-feed Evan a whole jar of pureed apple and some rice cereal for dinner, but only while he watched the show on the tablet. When Evan went to bed, Melissa and Dave had pressure cooked beef with vegetables. Melissa thought about saving some to send to daycare with Evan the next day, but figured he wouldn't eat any of it. Instead, she packed a couple of fruit pouches and baby crackers along with his bottles.

Evan's eating experiences are different from the rest of his family and are not as wholesome and enjoyable as they could be. He doesn't get opportunities to focus on the eating experience or to explore tastes and textures on his terms, which could enable him to progress to more complexity. His diet may be low in important nutrients. He doesn't have regular opportunities to eat meals with his parents and watch them enjoy whole foods.

Whether a baby grows into an adventurous, healthy eater depends on many factors. In the story above, Evan could be experiencing oral motor development or sensory processing challenges—or he might be developing typically. His early eating habits were shaped by his genetic predisposition and temperament, and will continue to be shaped by culture, his life experiences, and his overall health. When a baby joins your family, you don't know what kind of eater you'll have or what kinds of experiences await him later in life. But what you do during the first year matters.

Think about how many meals you will share with your child as he grows. Only a small fraction of them will happen during that short, but important, first year, when your baby has a tiny tummy and is growing and developing incredibly fast. And it's during these meals that you'll lay the foundation for his eating. The three building blocks of the optimal feeding environment are: (1) a setup for comfort and mastery, (2) nutrient-dense foods, and (3) responsive feeding.

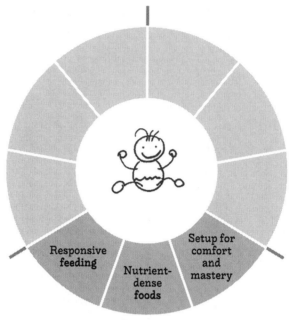

Feeding

The ONE approach: Universal building blocks for feeding.

The feeding environment you create shows your baby what food is and how to enjoy it in your family, your culture, and the world. An environment that offers delicious, nourishing foods while supporting mastery of eating skills in a responsive way will set your baby on the path to healthy and happy eating.

First nourishment: breastfeeding and formula-feeding

Your feeding relationship with your baby begins with milk. I hope that you feel supported and respected in your choices and your unique circumstances whether you feed your baby breast-milk, formula milk, or both.

Breastfeeding

If your baby is not here yet and you are planning to breastfeed, consider finding local breastfeeding support before you give birth: a lactation consultant, a midwife, a chapter of La Leche League, or some experienced and supportive women in your life. A study looked at mothers who gave birth in hospitals that actively supported breastfeeding and mothers who gave birth in hospitals that didn't actively support it, and found a striking difference in exclusive breastfeeding rates at three months: 43 percent compared to 6 percent.[165] Breastfeeding is natural, but it often takes time and effort to master. Having support when you have questions or concerns can make a big difference.

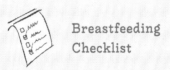

Breastfeeding
Checklist

Breastfeeding must-haves:
- ✓ Knowledge of where to turn if you need support
- ✓ A safe and comfortable place for night feedings

You might also like:
- ✓ A breast pump, a set of bottles (if you'll be expressing breastmilk and bottle-feeding)
- ✓ Breastmilk freezer bags
- ✓ A nursing pillow
- ✓ Breastfeeding-friendly clothes for you

The early days

Hold your baby skin-to-skin and offer her the breast as soon as possible after she's born to help smooth her transition into this world and to encourage your milk come in.[232] Your baby will likely be extra sleepy for the first day or so because of her high melatonin levels and her exhaustion from the birth itself. You should both use this time to rest.

Every time your baby wakes up (or more often, if advised by your baby's health care practitioner), bring her to your breast and encourage her to nurse as much as possible, giving her as much of the highly immune-supportive and protein-rich colostrum as you can. Observe your baby and tune into how you are feeling yourself so you can begin finding a comfortable nursing position. Make sure your body is well-supported and that you're leaning back: this will reduce tension in your shoulders, help you naturally support your baby's weight, and lead to better latch.[178] Gently support your baby's head and neck and make sure she's facing you, with her torso, neck, and head in a straight line. Follow her lead and feed her the way she wants to be fed. Let her eat as fast or as slowly as she wants; hold her quietly as she pauses or rests.[204]

Seeing You

Feeding is one of the few situations in which very young babies tend to keep their eyes open. The distance newborns can focus on best is about the distance from your breast to your face,[233] so if you feel like your baby is intently studying you, he probably is! Each feeding, now and later, is an opportunity to build and deepen your connection with your baby.

After that first sleepy day, most babies become more alert—and quite hungry. Many moms recall "the ravenous second night." It may seem like all you're doing is nursing, when you're so short on sleep. Still, try to nurse as much as you can: frequent feeding gives your baby that valuable colostrum and helps your milk come in.

Most women's milk comes on the third day (though, as mentioned earlier, it can range from 24 to 102 hours).[177] If your milk comes in quickly, you may experience engorgement as your breasts become full, tight, and sometimes painful. This is normal and will only last a few days as your body adjusts and settles into breastfeeding. The best way to feel more comfortable and to regulate your milk supply is to continue nursing whenever your baby wants.

How can you tell your baby is hungry? Look for these hunger clues:

- ✓ Increased alertness
- ✓ Turning her head to one side and seeming to "root" toward your breast
- ✓ Opening her mouth, sticking out her tongue, or puckering her lips

Crying is a *late* hunger sign. Once your baby starts crying, it may take a while for her to settle and feed well. Crying may also communicate other needs, such as tiredness, overwhelm, or discomfort. As you get to know your baby, you will learn to recognize her hunger cues more easily. When in doubt, offer your baby the breast to see if she's ready to feed.

Allow your baby to spend as much time at the breast as she wants to. The timing of the letdown (the milk ejection reflex), the speed of milk flow, and the milk's fat content differs from woman to woman; nursing style varies from baby to baby. Allowing your baby to feed for as long as she wants ensures that she takes in as much milk as she needs.

If you have concerns

Once your baby is actively feeding, you will notice a rhythm to the way she sucks, swallows, and breathes. If your baby "nipple feeds" (has only your nipple and little or no breast tissue in her mouth), frequently stops and pulls off, or makes clicking or "slurping" sounds, she is not latching well. Try adjusting your position: for example, lean back a bit more, bring your baby closer to your chest, and gently help her lips flare out if they are tucked under. If these adjustments are not helping, if you feel something isn't working quite right, and especially if you have concerns around your baby's weight gain or the number of wet diapers or if you're experiencing nipple pain or other persistent discomfort, talk to a lactation consultant or another trusted professional. These common issues don't necessarily mean that anything is wrong, but they are signs that you need extra support.

Tongue and lip ties (discussed on page 108) are common, but not always obvious. Figuring out whether your baby has a tie requires a close examination by an experienced professional. It is important to assess not only the tongue's appearance, but also its function.[234] Checking for ties is not always done at birth or during well-baby visits; there may or may not be routine screening where you live. In some countries lactation consultants can refer you to a specialist for assessment and surgical intervention; in others you'll need a referral from your family doctor or pediatrician. Don't stop if the initial advice you receive is conflicting; continue looking for help until you feel fully heard and supported. Your baby's and your own comfort and mastery are important.

As a new mom, you might worry about whether your baby is getting enough to eat. He most likely is, as longs as he's satisfied after his feedings and, after the first couple of days, produces plenty of wet and soiled diapers. Remember that breast size and fullness are not good indicators of milk supply, and neither is the length of your feedings because, as already mentioned, the letdown and milk flow rate differ from woman to woman and nursing style varies from baby to baby. Your health care team will monitor your baby's weight gain to be sure he's feeding and growing well. For the first couple of weeks, you may want to write down every time your baby feeds and has a wet or soiled diaper, so you have this information ready for the doctor visits.

Breastfeeding through the first year and beyond

Newborns and young babies often fall asleep at the end of a feeding. As your baby grows, consider working toward having him stay awake through most feedings. Being alert and calm will help your baby eat well, which will help you feel confident he's had enough to eat. This also allows you to burp him in the best position without worrying about waking him up. In addition, if your goal is independent sleep, your baby will have opportunities to practise self-settling if he goes to bed awake.

When your older baby is full, he may unlatch and turn away from the breast. One of my daughters did this from about five months on, clearly letting me know that she was done nursing. My other daughter, however, switched to slow, non-nutritive suckling: she would stay on the breast and move her jaw, but without the suck-swallow pattern of active nursing. Some babies have more need for such comfort-suckling than others. These babies are also more likely to use their fingers, thumb, or a pacifier for comfort and calming. If you offer your baby a pacifier, remember to introduce it after breastfeeding is established, and offer it mainly or only for sleep[191] and not for prolonged periods beyond the first year.[192]

Babies feed best when they are calm and comfortable. Once you master breastfeeding, you will likely find yourself feeding your baby in many spots in and out of your home. However, your baby will become more and more interested in her surroundings over time. Some babies are able to stay calm and focused when feeding regardless of what's going on around them, but others are easily distracted when fed in an unfamiliar place. (Remember, babies' brains are constantly looking for patterns and surprises). If your baby normally takes a full feed but begins "snacking" when distracted, she may benefit from having most of her feedings in a dedicated, calm space. You may want to use the space you set up for night feedings to feed your baby when you're home during the day. Make this space comfortable and cozy for your baby and for yourself.

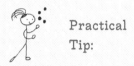

Practical
Tip:

If you have older children, you could include something special for them as you set up baby's feeding space. I put together a "special quiet basket" for Leah, who was a preschooler at the time, to explore when I was feeding Tessa; I included picture books, puzzles, and a photo book of Leah herself as a baby.

Continue with responsive breastfeeding: follow your baby's lead and feed him when you notice hunger cues. Trust that your baby is consuming exactly what he needs,[177,185] maintaining your milk supply.[186] If your baby's temperament is quite regular, you might settle into a rhythm where he generally feeds around the same times each day; just make sure that this rhythm is flexible and continues to be baby-led.

Your baby will have extra hungry days during his growth spurts; continue to follow his lead. Remember that most babies whose parents feed them responsively self-regulate how much they eat and grow just as they are supposed to.[185,202]

A string of hungry days does not necessarily mean a drop in your milk supply. Thinking "I don't have enough milk" is the most common reason mothers switch to formula or try to introduce solid foods early.[175,178] But if your mature milk has come in, your baby has a good latch, you've successfully established breastfeeding, and you are healthy, a big, irreversible drop in milk supply is quite rare. More common are these scenarios:

- Baby seems dissatisfied, fussy, and wakes up a lot at night— because her sleep is disorganized and she is overtired
- Baby is happy, but is taking much longer to nurse—because he is now comfort-suckling after feedings

In these scenarios, you may think you don't have enough milk, but as long as your baby is growing well, your milk supply is likely ample and consistent. When you find yourself worrying about supply, keep track of the number of wet diapers over the course of the day and check your baby's weight: see if he is following his usual trajectory. If he is, think about whether one of the above scenarios applies to you. Is your baby not getting enough sleep? Take a look at Chapter 2 for advice on how to help him—and yourself—become better rested. Is your baby nursing more frequently or for longer periods because of comfort-suckling? Decide whether you're comfortable with that or would like to stop feedings when your baby has finished nursing actively.

Last but not least, remember to eat well yourself and drink plenty of water. Aim to regularly include foods rich in omega-3s for your own health and to transfer omega-3s to your baby through breastmilk.[189]

Bottle-feeding breastmilk

Much of the advice above still applies if you bottle-feed expressed or donor milk. There are also a couple of additional considerations unique to bottle-feeding.

Some of the long-term benefits of breastfeeding have been attributed to the nurturing and close contact—the touching and gazing—breastfeeding provides.[168] Mothers and babies tend to touch and gaze at each other less during bottle-feeding compared to feeding from the breast.[233] But it doesn't have to be that way. When bottle-feeding, don't place your baby in an infant seat but cradle her against you, so she can see your face and feel your touch. (Reclining in a bucket-type infant seat is not the best feeding position anyway, because the shape of the seat tilts baby's pelvis and can put pressure on her esophagus.[235]) Although friends and extended family can help with bottle-feeding, your baby will likely eat best when fed by you or your partner: you know her and her hunger and fullness cues best, and she's most comfortable and relaxed with you.

Bottle-fed babies usually swallow more rapidly and drink faster than breastfeeding babies.[233] Bottle nipples also come in various sizes and milk flow speeds. To make sure the type you're using is a good fit for your baby, watch her feeding rhythm and overall comfort. If you see arching or squirming or don't see a steady suck-and-swallow rhythm, the milk is likely flowing too fast.

Bottle-fed babies play a less active role in feeding than those feeding from the breast because they don't have to work quite as hard at transferring the milk. But babies still know how much to drink from the bottle.[236] When you notice signs of your baby being full—slow, uninterested sucking or turning away from the bottle—offer the bottle a couple more times by gently touching baby's lips or cheek with the bottle nipple. Don't try to get your baby to finish the bottle: doing so may teach her to override her own internal sensation of being full.

It can be hard not to push the bottle if your baby was born prematurely, has been ill, or has colic. If you find yourself worrying about whether your baby takes enough milk, write down the amounts she drinks over the course of several days and talk to your baby's health care practitioner. They will check your baby's weight to see if she's following her normal growth trajectory.

Formula feeding

Formula-Feeding***
What You'll Need:

Must haves:

- ✓ Quality formula milk
- ✓ A set of bottles and nipples
- ✓ A safe and comfortable place for night feedings
- ✓ Knowledge of where to turn to if you need support

You might also choose:

- ✓ A bottle sterilizer
- ✓ A bottle warmer

Most cities have at least some breastfeeding support for new mothers, support that can be very helpful and sometimes even critical to feeding success. Interestingly, there is usually no dedicated support for parents who formula-feed. Yet it's important for formula-feeding families to find quality formula that suits their babies and to learn about responsive feeding. Rather than listening to sales and marketing people who represent specific brands, look for advice from a health care practitioner who's not associated with a formula company. Ask them for information about the products that are developed with the best available science in mind. At the time I write this in 2020, formulas enriched

---

*** You might notice that some of the text in this section repeats what was already covered in the "Bottle feeding breastmilk" section. I did this intentionally, to make sure that formula-feeding families who might have not read the previous section still had this information.

with omega-3 fatty acids and some prebiotics to support baby's microbiome are becoming available.[161, 194, 195] As research continues to move forward, new formula products may deliver even more functional benefits. If you have a family history of allergies, be sure to mention it to your baby's health care practitioner: some formulas are less likely to cause a reaction than others.

Set up a dedicated spot for feeding supplies, so you can easily see what you have and ensure everything is clean. Bottle nipples come in various sizes and milk flow speeds. To make sure the type you're using is a good fit for your baby, watch his feeding rhythm and overall comfort: is he feeding smoothly? Arching, squirming, and a lack of a steady suck-and-swallow rhythm are signs that the formula is flowing too fast. If you have questions, ask a lactation consultant to observe your baby feeding: lactation consultants are experienced in evaluating suck-and-swallow patterns, whether during breast or bottle feeding. Inspect bottle nipples frequently to make sure they're intact and replace them regularly.

Some of the long-term benefits of breastfeeding have been attributed to the nurturing and close contact—the touching and gazing—breastfeeding provides.[168] Mothers and babies tend to touch and gaze at each other less during bottle-feeding than during breastfeeding.[233] Yet, you absolutely can develop a close, nurturing feeding relationship when bottle-feeding formula. Cradle your baby against you so she can see your face and feel your touch. (Reclining in a bucket-type infant seat is not the best feeding position for babies, because the shape of the seat tilts baby's pelvis and can put pressure on the esophagus.[235]) Make sure your baby is comfortable so she can eat well. Gently support her head and neck in a way that aligns her head with her torso. Although friends and extended family can help with bottle-feeding, your baby will likely eat best when you or your partner feed her: you know her and her hunger and fullness cues best, and she's most comfortable and relaxed with you.

Your baby may benefit from having most feedings in a dedicated, calm space when you're home, especially as he gets older and becomes very interested in—and easily distracted by—what's going on around him. You may want to use the same space you set up for night feedings. Make this space comfortable and cozy for your baby and yourself.

Formula-fed babies have a less active role in feeding compared to those feeding from the breast, because they do not have to work quite as hard at transferring the milk. They also tend to show fewer hunger and fullness cues than breastfed babies.[237] But they still know how much to drink[236] and are able to consistently signal when they are full.[238, 239] It's common for babies to vary the amount of formula they take in from one feeding to another and from one day to the next, so try to follow your baby's cues in addition to watching the amount of formula in the bottle. When you notice signs of baby being full—slow, uninterested sucking, turning away from the bottle, or leaning away—offer the bottle a couple more times by gently touching her lips or cheek with the bottle nipple. Just check with her whether she had enough, don't try to get her to finish. Pushing the bottle may teach your baby to override her internal sensation of satiety and over time diminish her ability to feed to appetite.

It can be especially difficult to not push the bottle if your baby was born prematurely, has been ill, or has colic. If you find yourself worrying about whether your baby takes enough formula, record the amounts she drinks over the course of several days and talk to your baby's health care practitioner. They will check your baby's weight to see if she's following her normal growth trajectory.

Joining the family table: signs of readiness

Introducing solid foods is sometimes referred to as "weaning." This may sound like a taking-away process, but in fact it's quite the opposite. You are adding more nutrients and experiences with different foods while you continue to breastfeed, formula-feed, or both. Introducing your baby to the world of textures, aromas, and flavours is the beginning of a new phase that will last a lifetime: your son or daughter joining you at the family table.

As you prepare to introduce solid foods, consider not only how old your baby is, but also where he is developmentally: is he ready to play an active part in eating? Remember how wide the normal ranges are for motor skills and mealtime communication milestones (page 112). Your baby will likely be ready for solid foods sometime between four and six months when he can:[204]

- ✓ sit upright well, alone or with support
- ✓ open his mouth when he sees food coming
- ✓ close his mouth and turn his head away when he doesn't want it
- ✓ keep his tongue flat and low instead of pushing it out when something touches his lips (which tells us his tongue-thrust reflex has disappeared)

If your baby is younger than six months, healthy, and growing well, but not yet showing these signs, wait and keep observing. He's developing incredibly fast and there's a good chance he'll be ready as soon as next week.

From Your Baby's
Perspective:

Imagine you're at a restaurant. Your favourite dish is on the menu, yet you're offered another dish that looks quite unusual. You figure you'll give it a try. Except that you're told you must eat it while balancing on one foot and with one arm up in the air. How much would you be able to focus on the taste and texture of the dish? Would you enjoy it and look forward to trying it again?

This is how a baby who's not quite ready for solid food might feel.

Waking up more frequently at night is not, on its own, a sign that your baby needs solid food. Around four months, most babies begin waking more because of the changes in their sleep structure (see pages 74–76). Introducing solid foods does not help babies sleep better: babies fed solids are less likely to *feed* at night, but just as likely to *wake up*.[135] Try to keep your baby well-rested and wait until she's ready for solids.

What if your baby *is* showing signs of readiness, but doesn't have any teeth yet? You're good to go: she will be gumming, not chewing, her first foods anyway.

A setup for comfort and mastery

Just as with breast- and bottle-feeding, your baby will eat best when he's comfortable and calm. Don't use bucket-type "lounging" seats for feeding to avoid putting pressure on baby's esophagus.[235] Hold baby on your lap or use a feeding chair (high chair). Most feeding chairs are designed to last through toddlerhood, but that makes them much too wide for a little baby who's just starting on solids. There is, however, an easy way to make your baby more comfortable. Sit him upright in a high chair; add support around his hips, like a rolled up towel or receiving blanket, so he doesn't slump; and raise the footrest so his feet are supported. Another tip, offered by Nimali Fernando and Melanie Potock in *Raising a Healthy, Happy Eater*,[235] is to put a piece of spongy, waffle-weave shelf liner under your baby's bottom so he doesn't slide forward. Always make sure you can still safely buckle him in the chair as advised by the manufacturer. If your feeding chair reclines, don't feed your baby in a reclined position.

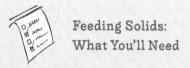

Feeding Solids: What You'll Need

✓ A feeding chair
✓ Two or three bibs (waterproof ones with a front pocket are especially handy)
✓ A set of soft wiping cloths
✓ A small open cup
✓ A small spoon (silicone or wood work well)

Choosing a Cup

Don't use sippy cups for too long; in fact, you can skip them entirely. Drinking from an open cup or a free-flow one without a valve encourages your baby to sip rather than suck, which helps his oral development.[192] Small silicone cups work well as they are easy to hold and don't break when dropped. Offer small sips of water from an open cup, free-flow cup, or a cup with a straw at every meal so your baby gets a bit of practice each time.

Purees and baby-led weaning

In deciding whether to start with purees or follow baby-led weaning (BLW), consider your baby's developmental readiness. Your baby may be ready for solids, but not yet ready to self-feed

BLW-style. Although some babies learn to grasp and self-feed pieces of food by six months, many are not ready until eight months or older.[197, 198, 211]

If you're starting with purees, you can begin with smoothly blended ones or slightly lumpy mashed ones, depending on your baby's readiness and your level of comfort. Either way, begin increasing texture at around six and a half or seven months to help with oral skills development.[149]

If you're starting with BLW, make sure all the foods you offer are a safe temperature, texture, shape, and size. Firm, round pieces about the size of baby's airway are choking hazards. Don't give your baby hard foods that can snap off and leave a chunk in his mouth—not even to just explore or hold. A good BLW food is one that is easily mashed when pushed against the roof of the mouth with a tongue: for example, a well-cooked, soft, thin stick of vegetable or fruit. To make sure the temperature and texture are right, try it yourself first.

An Important Word on Safety

Gagging and choking are not the same thing. Gagging is a normal and necessary reflex that keeps food well to the front of the mouth and prevents large pieces from being swallowed; it is nature's way of protecting the airway and is very common in babies learning to eat. Choking, however, is a life-threatening medical emergency when the airway becomes obstructed. It is possible to choke on soft food. Unlike gagging, choking is usually silent.

Regardless of the feeding style you choose, always stay within arm's reach and watch your baby closely during all feedings, with absolutely no exceptions. Never give your baby snacks when she's strapped in a car seat, not even soft squeezable pouches of baby food. Don't let older babies crawl or walk with food in their mouths. Learn the Heimlich manoeuvre and CPR for babies and children.[240]

There are several full-length books written specifically on BLW. However, in my opinion, there's actually not that much difference between BLW and the traditional spoon-feeding route. In both methods, you can set aside foods from your family meals that are appropriate for baby. In both methods, you have the opportunity to offer your baby a variety of flavours and to progress to more complex textures and tastes. And, importantly, *both feeding styles are, in fact, baby-led, as long as you tune in and feed responsively.* I chose spoon-feeding for my children; I saw it as a short phase that led to competent self-feeding. Many families combine feeding styles right from the start. They offer their babies both purees from a spoon and pieces of food to self-feed. Either way, nutritious foods and responsive feeding are key.

Cooking nutrient-dense foods: a stage-by-stage guide

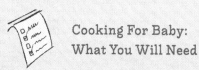

Cooking For Baby:
What You Will Need

✓ A stainless steel or cast iron cooking pot with a steamer insert
✓ A roasting pan
✓ A hand-held blender
✓ An ice cube tray (one with a lid works best)

You probably have some or even all of these items in your kitchen already. This is all you need. These simple tools are just as functional as specialized "baby food systems" that are expensive but useful only for a short time.

From first bites to eight months: simple tastes

Here's what you can do for your baby's first tastes of solid foods:

✓ Select baby-friendly foods from the family meal: Set aside a well-cooked steamed or roasted vegetable from your meal (for example, peas, carrot, squash, or sweet potato) and puree or mash it for the baby, adding a bit of breastmilk, formula, or cooking water.

✓ Cook something especially for your baby: Steam or poach a piece of fruit (such as pear, apple, or peach) or bake or steam a vegetable (carrot, squash, yam, sweet potato) until it's well-cooked and soft; puree it, mash it, or cut it into thin strips.

✓ Offer ready-to-serve nutrient-dense foods: Use naturally soft fruits (avocado, banana, very ripe pear or peach), peeled and pureed or mashed.

You will likely use a combination of these approaches in the first few weeks as your baby gets accustomed to solid food. I like to think of it as *supportive and simple meal planning.* To support your baby, choose foods that are nutrient-dense, tasty, and have texture that your baby can process with ease. This will help your baby feel more comfortable and confident in her eating, encouraging mastery. To make feeding simple and sustainable for yourself, include baby-friendly foods in your regular meals as much as possible so you don't have to cook separately for your baby. (Nutrient-dense foods are good for you, too!)

Should you introduce one food at a time? Most pediatricians agree that for babies without a family history of allergies, foods can be introduced safely without following a particular schedule, adding one food at a time, or waiting a certain number of days before introducing a new food. You might want to introduce one food at a time if allergies do run in your family or if your baby develops signs that point to food sensitivities, such as skin rashes or constipation.

Foods You Should Not Give Your Baby

✗ Honey

✗ Cow's milk

✗ Unpasteurized foods

✗ Nutrient-poor, processed foods high in saturated fats, sugar, or salt

✗ Choking hazards: Any foods that are firm and round and foods that could separate into firm and round pieces

---

Begin incorporating iron-rich foods early and serve them often. Here are some ideas for making it easier:

- High-iron foods like meats, egg yolks, and fish can be tough or dry in texture for young babies to comfortably eat. Puree them with gravy or vegetables to soften and moisten the meat.

- Add cooked and mashed or pureed beans or lentils to vegetable purees.

- Mix iron-fortified infant cereals into vegetable or fruit purees.

Talk to your baby's health care practitioner about the need for vitamin or mineral supplements. They will make recommendations based on where you live, your family's eating style, and your baby's nutritional status.

Offer solid foods after breastmilk or formula, and when your baby is alert and content. Begin with two meals a day and increase the number of meals following your baby's appetite and interest. Naps already structure your baby's day; add meals to the windows of time when your baby is well-rested and alert.

Practical Tips on Adding Nutrients,
Healthy Fats, and Flavour:

✓ Boost flavour in vegetables by sautéing or roasting them in olive oil.

✓ Make a pot of chicken, beef, or beef bone broth (grass-fed beef and marrow bones make the best broth); strain it, cool it, pour it into an ice cube tray, and freeze. Thaw it in the fridge one cube at a time and add it to foods that you're mashing or pureeing for your baby.

✓ Set aside meat and vegetables from your meal and mash or puree them using a hand-held blender with a bit of broth, olive oil, or gravy; puree them when they're hot, so the fat can melt through, but be sure to let them cool before serving.

✓ Use in-season, locally grown, organic fruits and vegetables as much as possible: they are more nutrient-dense and more flavourful.

You will soon find a feeding rhythm that fits with the overall rhythm of the day. For example, feeding times of a seven-month-old baby might look like this:

A Four-Nap Day
6:45 a.m.: wake up, breastmilk or formula
7:30 a.m.: breakfast
8:45–10:05 a.m.: first nap, breastmilk or formula before and after
11 a.m.: lunch
12:30–3:00 p.m.: second nap, breastmilk or formula before and after
5 p.m.: dinner
6:00 p.m.: breastmilk or formula, bedtime

Eight months and beyond: more complexity and independence

Your older baby has now experienced a variety of flavours and is becoming more skilled in self-feeding. He can now eat most of the foods in the family meals, mashed or cut into small pieces. Continue with supportive and simple meal planning. Your baby may enjoy the flavours of spices and herbs, but if you like your food very spicy, consider separating out the baby's portion first before adding strong spices or hot sauce.

Most families introduce snacks around the end of the first year. It's somewhat easy to fall into the nutrient-poor snack trap: snacks are often eaten on the go, and it's convenient to offer a packaged, high-sugar item. But a poor-quality snack robs your child twice: once when he eats it and again when the calories replace those of a more nutritious meal to be served later.[204] I like to think of snacks as mini-meals, rather than treats. I know that you're not going to offer your baby treats like candy in the first year, but it's important to start thinking about this idea of seeing snacks as small meals early on, so it becomes second-nature as your baby grows. In the first year, the simplest approach to snacks is to refrigerate an extra serving of food from your baby's breakfast or lunch for a snack later that day.

Responsive feeding

Our role in feeding

Every feeding is an opportunity for learning and connection. Babies are born with strong capabilities to like new foods and to eat to their appetite, but they need our support to retain these capabilities.

What does this mean in practice? I find Ellyn Satter's approach,[204] mentioned on page 114, most helpful:

- Parents and other caregivers set up a nurturing feeding environment and provide nutritious foods
- Babies decide how much of each food to eat and whether to eat it at all

Our role is to create a supportive feeding environment and then trust our babies to eat as much as they need. In other words, we put effort into what we offer and not into "making" babies eat.

Responsive spoon-feeding

Christian is about to feed seven-month-old Ella lunch. He notices that she looks tired and is rubbing her eyes. Remembering that her morning nap was very short, he gives her a bottle and puts her down for a nap first. When she wakes up, he changes her diaper and tells her it is time for lunch. He picks her up and positions her in the feeding chair, making sure she's comfortably sitting upright, and then sits down facing her. Ella looks a bit impatient, but Christian has already prepared a small serving bowl with vegetables mashed with a well-cooked egg yolk, a small open cup with water, a spoon, a bib, and a cloth. He tells Ella what food is in the bowl, scoops up a small amount and brings it close to her. She looks at the food for a little while, then slowly opens her mouth and tastes it. She makes a funny face as if the food is sour, but then stretches out her arms and opens her mouth for more. Christian keeps feeding her until she stops opening her mouth eagerly and begins playing with the spoon instead. He offers Ella water by bringing the cup to her lips; she takes a couple of sips as he holds the cup. Christian then tells Ella he is going to clean up, and that she can explore the spoon for a bit.

Responsive self-feeding

Eleven-month-old Rylan is exploring "his" shelf in the kitchen; he's figuring out how to fit measuring spoons into a cup. Katie has prepared his lunch—chicken, squash, and avocado, cut into small pieces—and her own lunch of chicken and avocado salad. She waits a moment until Rylan looks at her, then she tells him it's time for lunch and that she's going to pick him up. She positions him in the high chair and sits down beside him with a small serving bowl for Rylan and her own lunch. She places a couple of pieces of each food on the high chair tray while telling Rylan what the foods are. Rylan eats the squash right away— it's one of his favourites—and Katie adds some more to the tray. He tries the chicken next. Katie eats her lunch and keeps adding more food to Rylan's tray, a few pieces at a time. Rylan tries to pick up the avocado, but it's too slippery for him to grasp; he pushes the pieces off the tray and onto the floor. Noticing that, Katie mashes a small piece of avocado and offers him some on a spoon. Rylan turns away and begins moving the remaining pieces of food around the tray. Katie offers him one more piece of squash, asks him if he's all done, and puts the food away. Rylan drinks some water from a straw cup and stretches his arms up, eager to get out of the high chair. Katie wipes his face and hands as Rylan helps by holding the cloth.

Note how both Christian and Katie:

- Kept their attention on their babies
- Described what they were doing and what foods they were offering
- Put a small amount of food in front of their babies, enough to interest them but not so much that it might overwhelm them or invite them to play with it
- Gave their babies time to use their senses of sight, smell, and taste at their own pace
- Continued offering more food a little at a time, watching their babies' interest and appetite, making the meal feel like a conversation

- Waited for their babies to communicate their satiety
- Did not limit the amount of food or push for more

Ella and Rylan both had an opportunity to enjoy the food, to experience mealtime as a time for connection, and to feel their parents' support.

Try not to feed your baby as a way to comfort her when she's tired or upset. Using food for its main purpose—to satisfy hunger through nutrition—allows your baby to keep her innate capability to eat to appetite. Observe your baby carefully and respond to her sensitively: comfort her when she's upset, feed her when she's hungry. This helps reaffirm her sensations and feelings and builds trust, connection, and communication. This will continue being important as your baby grows into an older child and even into adulthood.

Exploring tastes takes time and patience

Continue offering foods that your baby initially rejects. Remember, he may need eight or more tastes, in different meals and in a supportive, no-pressure setting before he accepts the new flavour.[212, 213] In the example above, Katie might choose to continue offering Rylan some avocado every time she eats it herself. Although nothing guarantees that Rylan will love avocadoes when he grows up, there is a very good chance that after several tastes, avocadoes will become part of his diet.

It can be upsetting when your baby rejects food, especially when it's a special meal you enjoyed cooking. But don't try to coerce your baby to eat it. Instead, simply save the extras to try later that day or, if it's something that freezes well, puree and freeze it in an ice cube tray. (However, always discard any leftovers from the serving bowl itself for food safety: the baby's saliva mixed with the unused food can feed harmful bacteria.) Once extra food is frozen, transfer the cubes into a re-sealable freezer bag, then thaw them in the fridge a few at a time when you want to offer the food again.

Give your baby plenty of opportunities to experiment and master eating. When you see him putting food in his mouth and taking it back out, it's a good thing: he's tasting it, and therefore building those eight or more tastes he might need to learn to like it. Making "funny" faces during eating is not necessarily a sign of dislike either: your baby simply has very sensitive taste buds! Some exploring of food is good, too, as it helps your baby engage all his senses and learn about the joy of eating. However, playing with food or throwing is usually a sign of a baby being full.

> *When your baby puts food in his mouth and takes it back out, it's a good thing: he's tasting it, building up experiences he might need to learn to like it.*

Eating together

Your baby is learning a lot through the positive, repeated experiences with healthy foods. He's also learning by seeing others—and especially you—enjoy eating. Share meals with your baby whenever possible to model healthy, happy eating. Eating together will take longer than eating on your own; plan for this and try to enjoy the process as much as the outcome.

A feeding story

My daughters' eating journeys are very similar, so I'll share one of them.

I breastfed Tessa exclusively for the first six months. Following our physician's advice, she also received a daily dose of liquid vitamin D. At five and a half months, Tessa was sitting well independently and looked at food with interest when others were eating. One day, I set up her feeding chair, made sure she was comfortable, and put her usual drop of vitamin D on a spoon, rather than on the nipple before nursing. Tessa pushed the spoon out with her tongue, showing me that she still had the tongue-thrust reflex. I tried again in a week, and this time she didn't push it out. It looked like she was ready for solids.

So, at just under six months old Tessa had her first taste of solid food: some roasted sweet potato. I chose to start with smooth purees with the goal of gradually encouraging Tessa to progress to mashed textures and small pieces.

During the following month we introduced a variety of meats and well-cooked root vegetables (yam, carrot, parsnip, squash) and fruits (banana, peach, cooked apple and pear, plum). For the most part, these foods came from our family dinners. I experimented with flavours by poaching apples with dried apricot, pears with a tiny bit of ginger, and plums with dried figs. I chose organic, locally grown fruits and vegetables as much as possible. For iron and energy, I put infant oatmeal and a drop of unsulfured, pasteurized blackstrap molasses into fruit purees; I added small amounts of whole grains (quinoa and buckwheat), chicken and beef broth, and olive oil to vegetables. Tessa also enjoyed sardines mashed into potato puree. She ate a trusted brand of store-bought baby food when we travelled.

At seven months, Tessa developed a rash after eating egg yolk, and again after eating a bit of butter, so I didn't feed her eggs or dairy for several months. I gave her a good quality infant probiotic recommended by our physician during this time. (She eats these foods now and is not allergic or sensitive to them.)

I enjoy cooking, so I made some meals especially for Tessa. I highly recommend the book Wholefood for Children[241] by Jude Blereau for meal ideas and recipes if you love cooking. Tessa's *favourite full-meal combinations, inspired by Blereau's recipes, included:*

- *Red lentils cooked in chicken broth with butternut squash and dark leafy greens*
- *Local fish cooked in vegetable stock and coconut milk with carrot and green peas*

By about nine months, Tessa was mostly eating the same foods as the rest of our family, mashed or cut into small pieces. She had days where she was ravenous and adventurous in her eating and days when she didn't eat as much, but overall she has always enjoyed eating and trying new foods. She continued to breastfeed until she was twenty months old.

Questions you may have

Q I really wanted to breastfeed my first child, but I couldn't. I am anxious about whether I'll be able to breastfeed my new baby.

A Try to pinpoint the reason that breastfeeding didn't work the first time. Successful breastmilk production requires three things: sufficient glandular tissue in the breast, normal hormone levels, and regular removal of milk. Some issues and conditions cannot be resolved (for example, breast hypoplasia, a rare situation where glandular tissue in the breast is not sufficient to support breastfeeding[242]) but these are uncommon. Most women can produce enough milk with proper support.

If you weren't able to breastfeed because of a certain medication you were taking, share your concerns with your health care practitioner and ask about alternatives.

Challenges on baby's side, such as latching difficulties or persistent thrush, won't necessarily be present in your second baby even if they were for the first. If you do encounter them again, they, too, can usually be resolved with proper support. Map out lactation support available in your area; if you can, talk to a lactation consultant or another trusted, experienced professional before your new baby arrives. Most importantly, be gentle with yourself.

Q **My baby is seven months old and refuses solids. I've tried many types of commercial and homemade baby foods. She spits everything right out. I don't know what to do.**

A Continue offering solid foods two or three times a day and continue breast- or formula-feeding on demand. Offer foods when your baby is alert, content, and not too tired. Try experimenting with textures: if you've been trying smooth purees so far, try a slightly more lumpy consistency or cut very soft vegetables or fruits into sticks. If your baby is having fewer wet and soiled diapers than before or you have concerns about her nutritional status or behaviour, be sure to see her health care practitioner.

Q **I am going back to work. How can I best support my baby's eating while I'm away from him?**

A If a nanny or a family member will be caring for your baby, talk to them about your approaches to feeding. Ask them to read this book or parts of it. Write down your baby's usual feeding times. Ask them to watch you feeding your baby.

If your baby will be in a daycare centre, discuss the centre's approaches to feeding before you enrol. Does the centre provide some or all of the food? Ask what the typical meals are and how they're served. Make sure all the foods provided by the centre or sent from home are nutritious and have the texture and shape your baby can process with ease.

Touch base with your baby's main caregiver every day when you pick him up to find out how he ate.

Watch and Wonder

During a night feeding, feel the quiet, the warmth, and the closeness. Some time soon your baby will stop feeding at night. The feeding the night before that will become the very last one; you won't know it until later, and you may never be able to pinpoint the exact date. But you will forever remember how it felt.

Every feeding is an opportunity for learning and love. There will be times when you feel tired or rushed. Remember that tomorrow will be a new day.

Make a video of your baby's first time eating solid foods, even if nothing ends up being actually eaten. Record what the very first food was, because one day your child will ask.

Remember that you cannot (and should not) make your baby eat. You are responsible for feeding—providing nutritious food and a safe place and appropriate time to eat—but it is your baby who's responsible for eating.

In the next chapter, we'll look into the science of child development and how it can help us create environments for connection, play, and exploration.

CHAPTER 4
CARE AND PLAY

Most parents want their children to be prepared as they step into the fast-paced outside world that's teeming with choices and opportunities. So we pass young babies around for others to hold so they become more social. We buy expensive educational toys and enrol our babies in enrichment activities. However, approaches we consider natural, normal, or optimal are not necessarily such. All too often they are simply *common* and culturally approved: everyone around us is doing things a certain way, so we do the same. And sometimes these practices in fact conflict with babies' biology and don't support their natural development. Let's take a look at what the science says.

PART I
INFANT DEVELOPMENT

"Young children are very busy. Their evolution ... makes what we do as adults look like standing still"
—Kim John Payne, *Simplicity Parenting*

What babies accomplish in their first year is truly astounding. Imagine arriving to a new planet with different laws of physics and proceeding to learn a new language or two, fall in love, figure out a new culture, and master at least five different sports, all in one year. Babies do the equivalent of this and more.

Parents often notice periods of rapid change when their baby's new abilities emerge.[20] You might have heard of these periods as developmental shifts, transitions, or "wonder weeks." But for any new ability to become integrated and eventually dominant and visible to us, much development unfolds gradually and constantly behind the scenes. Our babies are always working hard.

What Is Baby Working On?

- **Birth to 3 months:** Adjusting inner rhythms and states to the environment;[20] staying calm and regulated
- **2 to 3 months:** Focusing; detecting emotional expressions of others
- **3 to 5 months:** Developing physical mobility; organizing sleep

- *5 to 7 months:* Understanding that people and objects exist even when they're not immediately present (object permanence); eating solid foods
- *7 to 9 months:* Building focused attachment (different responses to primary caregivers); learning to detect patterns and anticipate events;[25] understanding words and placing them into categories
- *9 to 12 months:* Expanding physical mobility; understanding other people's behaviours and preferences
- *12 months and on:* Becoming more independent; exploring limits

These are some of the major transitions, skills, and milestones babies are working on at each stage, but there are many other things they are discovering and learning.

At each stage, babies get better at mastering and integrating previous skills and begin working on ones that come after. And through all stages, babies are simultaneously developing along three major strands: social-emotional, cognitive, and sensory and motor. Let's take a look at these three developmental strands and then examine how you can take them into account as you care for your baby in your home and out in the wider world.

Social-emotional development

Social-emotional development refers to a baby's growing ability to experience, express, and manage emotions and establish relationships with others. In supportive environments babies gradually get better and better at:

- Expecting safety and support from family and other caregivers
- Communicating their needs and feelings
- Understanding their own emotions and the emotions of others
- Carrying forward a sense of competence and trust[20]

Mastering these skills is not an easy feat, and most of us continue to learn and improve through adulthood. Let's explore how and when babies begin learning about emotions, actions, and words, and what we can do to help.

Understanding emotions, actions, and words

Babies come into the world ready to connect and learn. You might recall from Chapter 1 that newborns can tell if someone is looking at them or away from them.[15] Even one-month-old babies can perceive facial expressions; if a parent assumes a sombre, still face showing no emotion, baby's heart activity changes in a distinct way that indicates distress and active coping. This means babies sense their parents' support and learn to rely on it very early on.[243, 244]

Two-month-old babies can anticipate actions that they see and experience regularly. When adults approach babies to pick them up in a way that is slow and clearly visible, babies adjust their posture to help with the smoothness of the pickup: they focus on the adult's face, tense their neck and back muscles, and open their arms a little wider, creating space for the adult's hands. Even at this young age babies are able to participate in a joint intentional routine in a meaningful way—but only if the adult's intentions are clear and visible.[54, 245]

Five-month-olds are beginning to extract individual words from speech, usually starting with their own name.[246, 247] Although they can hear almost as well as adults at this point, they are disadvantaged when there is background noise:[248] because their ears and brains treat all sound input the same way, they find it harder to separate out individual words when speech is masked by other sounds.

Young babies cannot yet understand what people are talking about, so it's hard for them to detect when someone is addressing them—much like it is for foreigners![247] To help with that, adults and older children around the world tend to intuitively change the way they speak when talking to babies: they make eye contact, call the baby by name, position themselves face-to-face, slow down, and talk using short sentences, often in a singsong voice.[249] When adults look at babies and talk to them this way, babies show enhanced brain activation.[247] This tells us that babies know when they're being talked to—and when they are, they work hard to process the communication. It doesn't mean that we must be overly animated or always use a high-pitched voice, as some suggest. But helping babies understand that we're talking to them, through eye contact and body language, helps them tune in to communicating with us.

By six months, babies understand a number of common nouns and are beginning to put words into categories.[250] Learning words requires matching sounds with objects or events they represent, so repeatedly hearing words in context ("Look at the rain!") helps babies learn them. It is especially beneficial when parents notice what babies are interested in and label these objects or events: it helps babies relate what they're looking at with the words they're hearing.[250]

Amazingly, six-month-olds can already tell helpful and hindering behaviours apart. In a series of neat experiments, babies were shown a puppet—a simple shape with googly eyes—that was trying to climb a hill (the "climber"). After the initial attempt, another puppet either helped it by pushing it up from behind or hindered by pushing it down the hill. When offered to explore the puppets, six-month-olds invariably reached for the "helper" and not the "hinderer"! This suggests that six-month-olds may be able to assess individuals based on their behaviour toward others, the early groundwork for moral thinking.[251]

At ten months, babies still preferred the "helper," but also looked at the puppets for considerably longer if, after the climb, the "climber" moved over to sit with the "hinderer" instead of the "helper." Babies were surprised by this behaviour because it was different from what they expected (why would anyone want to be with someone who was not nice to them?). At six months such behaviour did not yet surprise babies. This suggests that ten-month-olds are able to not only make their own assessment of someone else's behaviour, but also grasp other people's evaluation of each other.[251]

By six months babies learn to perceive facial expressions, anticipate actions they see and experience regularly, recognize their names and a number of other common words, and even recognize whether behaviours of others are helpful or unhelpful.

Twelve-month-olds are able to read their parents' emotional expressions and change their own behaviour accordingly. In one experiment, babies were invited to cross a drop-off in the ground to explore the other side; the drop-off was covered with plexiglass, so crossing was completely safe, but it may not have appeared that way to them. When their moms showed joy or interest, babies crossed confidently; if their moms showed fear or anger, they retreated; and if their mothers appeared sad, they stopped at the edge and kept looking across the space.[252] They trusted and followed their moms' emotional signals when the signals were clear.

What we do and how we do it affects how babies understand themselves and the social world they live in. But what matters most of all? Not surprisingly, science says it's our relationships with our babies.

What matters most for social-emotional development

According to the theory of attachment, most important for healthy social-emotional development is a close, committed relationship with one or more adults.[36, 37] As you may recall from Chapter 1, secure attachment comes from the quality of the relationship—the strong and mutual emotional connection—rather than specific techniques. The adults become baby's secure base as she develops *basic trust*: a positive attitude toward herself and the world that is formed early in life.[253]

When your baby grows into an older child and eventually into an adult, how would you want her to react to emotionally intense situations, whether exciting or stressful ones? Many parents want their children to experience emotions, but not be overwhelmed by them; to get excited, but not frenetic; to feel enough anxiety to be careful, but not so much as to become overly worried or avoid emotional experiences altogether. In other words, we want our children to be able to recognize their emotions and find a balanced way to manage them. It is important to know that the process of emotional regulation begins during babyhood.

Baby's ability to adjust the environment to fit his emotional state is very limited. For example, when a baby feels overwhelmed, he can try avoiding further stimulation by turning away or falling asleep; he could also try self-comforting by, for example, sucking his thumb.[20, 41] But for the most part he requires a caring adult to meet his needs: in this example, notice his distress and gently take him to a quieter environment or offer him a nap. When baby's needs are met consistently, he develops secure attachment and learns trust. His nervous system learns to regulate intense emotions more flexibly: as he practises shifting between different states, staying calm and returning to a calm state becomes easier for him. In other words, the baby-parent relationship across the first year affects a baby's capacity for emotional regulation on a physiological level:[41] his body begins to handle emotions in a more balanced way when he's supported by, and securely attached to, his parents and other committed caregivers in his life.

The baby-parent relationship during the first year affects baby's physiological capacity to regulate emotions.

Secure attachment forms best when parents and caregivers show sensitivity and mind-mindedness,[26,39] which I mentioned briefly in Chapter 1. Let's take a closer look.

Sensitivity

Sensitivity is a way of *being with babies* and *responding to them*. It reflects the adult's ability to perceive, accurately interpret, warmly accept, and respond to baby's signals.[254] Responsiveness—the way we respond to our babies' needs—is sometimes thought of simply as promptness. When the instructor in our prenatal class asked, "How should you respond to your baby?" all of us said in unison "Right away!" Indeed, in the early studies on attachment, researchers noticed that mothers of securely attached babies tended to respond promptly.[255] But later on it was shown that *adequacy of response* is just as important, and sometimes more important, than promptness.[28,256] A response is adequate when it is well-matched to the baby's needs, emotions, and developmental level, as well as to the particular situation.[26]

From Your Baby's
Perspective:

Imagine you're at a crowded party. You're trying to tell a friend that you would like to step outside for a minute to take a break, but she hands you the karaoke microphone to "cheer you up." This response is prompt, but will probably not feel adequate to you.

A tired baby whose well-meaning parents are shaking a rattle to distract him might feel this way.

Sensitivity is particularly important when babies are upset or communicating other immediate needs. How parents respond teaches babies about emotional states and about what they might expect from others. Babies can learn from a very early age to perceive the expression and sharing of "negative" emotions as acceptable: they can learn that all emotions are valuable and worthy of response. When parents respond sensitively and consistently, their babies tend to grow into toddlers with fewer behavioural problems and greater social competence, regardless of the temperaments they were born with; moreover, babies with more intense temperaments often begin showing distress less intensely as they grow.[26]

Sensitivity is still important when babies are content and exploring happily. A parent or caregiver observing a baby's play sensitively has an opportunity to notice and support the baby's interests in the moment, instead of interrupting, distracting, or re-directing. In the scientific literature this approach is called "supporting baby's focus of attention." Doing so encourages babies to take a more active role in play and social interactions as they grow. When mothers respond sensitively, support babies' focus of attention, and use rich language as they label objects that babies show interest in, babies tend to cooperate better during daily routines, use words more, and play independently for longer periods of time in their second year. They also use toys in more complex ways, showing greater problem-solving skills.[256]

Mind-mindedness

Mind-mindedness is a tendency to view babies as people with minds of their own.[39, 257] This concept is related to sensitivity, but captures a slightly different aspect:[258] while sensitivity is a way of being with babies and responding to them, mind-mindedness is a way of *thinking* about babies.

Parents who recognize that babies have their own sensations, emotions, and thoughts tend to be more insightful. They adjust their views and practices as they watch their babies, instead of relying on their own wishes or general ideas of what a baby needs or should be doing.[40] They are able to see things from their baby's perspective.[39] They also tend to comment on what their baby might be thinking and feeling. Remember that babies begin understanding and categorizing words by around six months old? When parents label emotions, babies learn about emotions and begin recognizing them.[41, 259] Studies show that babies who grow in mind-minded environments tend to develop stronger bonds with their parents, learn to speak earlier, and understand the emotions and needs of others around them better.[42, 43]

Mind-mindedness comes from within the parent and can be learned and practised intentionally[38] regardless of a baby's temperament,[39, 41] age, or developmental stage. Chapter 1 offered you advice on how to practice mind-mindedness before your baby arrives and in the very early days with your baby (pages 16–19). In Part II of this chapter, I will show you how to continue practising mind-mindedness as your baby grows.

Together, sensitivity and mind-mindedness create conditions for strong attachment: baby communicates, parent responds in a sensitive and mind-minded way, and baby experiences her needs being met, her emotions accepted, and her interests supported in a warm and predictable way. Baby's brain forms positive expectations about the social and emotional world around her, giving her a secure home base. She develops a sense of trust and safety, and is free to explore and learn.

Cognitive development

Cognitive development refers to a baby's growing and changing mental abilities: thinking, reasoning, and understanding. During the first year babies gradually get better at gathering and organizing information, remembering, problem solving, and predicting events. To do so, they use universal learning methods that closely resemble scientific research.

How babies learn

At the core of any learning is the ability to pay attention and notice new things. To fully notice something, one must detect something new, separate it from everything else, make sense of it, and store it in memory. As babies grow, everything they notice—their observations—gradually accumulate and construct their knowledge of the world.

Much like scientists, babies place events they have repeatedly observed into categories, and then they use these categories to predict the outcomes of future events. For example, by about five months a baby usually learns that when she drops something, it falls down.[49] It will take her years to label this as gravity, but she's discovered a pattern about her physical surroundings:

Observation + Observation + Observation = Pattern

Next time baby sees something dropped, she is not surprised: her brain tags this predicted experience as "usual," integrates it into existing knowledge, and stops paying attention to it. But when her experience is unusual—for example, she sees a helium balloon that floats instead of falling—she cannot easily fit this observation into her existing knowledge. Because of this, her brain pays special attention.[260]

Across many studies, babies have been shown to respond in a certain way when their expectations are not met: they look for longer[261] and show different brain activity. For example, in recent experiments eleven-month-olds who saw an object defy their expectations paid more attention and explored the object more.[262] Moreover, they tested theories relevant to the object's behaviour: when they were given a ball they had previously seen rolling off an edge, but not falling, they repeatedly dropped it; when they saw a ball seemingly pass through a solid wall, they repeatedly banged it on the floor.[262] These babies used the conflict between predicted and observed behaviour to gain knowledge about the world:

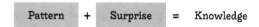

Pattern   +   Surprise   =   Knowledge

Observing and learning patterns gives babies a beginning sense of physics and mathematics. As mentioned earlier, by five months babies have an understanding that unsupported objects fall.[49] They begin understanding that liquids and solids behave differently around six months,[263] and they gain a sense of object transparency around eight or nine months.[261]

Patterns and surprises continue to be driving forces for learning well beyond babyhood. You will have many opportunities to see pattern-based reasoning in the future, like when your toddler proudly announces "I eated!"

Brain growth and development

You have undoubtedly heard that early childhood is an extremely important period for brain development. A newborn's brain is her least developed organ, at only a quarter of its adult size. Her total brain volume will double in the first year and reach 80 to 90 percent of its adult size by the time she's two years old.[264] But it's not only growth that matters; it's also what happens inside the brain.

The part of the human brain that's responsible for intelligence, language, memory, and creativity—our most important mental capacities—is called the neocortex. Very recently, researchers proved what they had suspected for many years: no neurons are added to the neocortex after birth. In other words, all of the brain cells composing the neocortex are formed before a baby is born and are retained for his entire life.[265-267] The human brain develops not by adding new cells, but by *creating and re-organizing connections* within itself.[267]

> ### The Importance of Environment for Human Brain Development
>
> The human brain consists of billions of neurons and is wired by approximately 20,000 genes. This may sound like a lot, but a strikingly similar number of genes has been discovered in a small worm with only 302 neurons. How, then, do human behaviour and cognitive abilities develop so far beyond those of a worm? It happens because genes provide only general developmental signals for the human brain: a blueprint, a rough framework. The environment—the experiences each person has—drives brain construction.[268] Essentially, our minds are fine-tuned to our environment.

Childhood is recognized as the most crucial stage for development because this is when the majority of brain wiring happens. As babies experience life outside the womb, billions of cells are wired into interconnected networks, layers, columns, and functional areas in a process called *blooming*. During blooming, babies' brains become more highly connected than they will be in adulthood, with more neural pathways. A typical two-year-old has at least twice the number of brain connections she will have when she grows up.

Each connection begins as relatively weak. Over time connections that are used more get strengthened,[269, 270] while those that are used less are gradually eliminated in a process called *pruning*. Pruning in the sensory cortex—the area of the brain that processes input from hearing, sight, and other senses—begins as early as eight months.[271] In other brain areas most pruning takes place between five years old and puberty, and then the number of connections stabilizes at adult levels that are maintained until old age.[272] As Dr. Alison Gopnik describes in *The Philosophical Baby*, babies' brains look like a map of old Paris, with many winding, interconnected little streets; in contrast, adult brains have fewer but more efficient boulevards and even highways.[273]

Does this mean we should choose intense enrichment activities for our babies and toddlers so they grow *more* connections during the blooming phase of brain development? Science says no.[269, 271, 274, 275] The number of brain connections appears to be largely under genetic control. Blooming can get disrupted in extreme circumstances like malnutrition, toxin exposure, and chronic stress,[269, 271] but under normal circumstances babies' experiences do not affect the number of brain connections. In other words, deprivation disrupts blooming, but enrichment does not enhance it. However, experiences do affect connection *strength*, determining which connections stay and which ones get pruned out. So what matters is not *how much* baby is exposed to, but *what* the events or activities are and *how* she experiences them. This is why early experiences are important.

> *The number of brain connections we have is largely determined by genetics, but experiences affect connection strength. Because of this, what the events or activities are and how baby experiences them matter more than how much baby is exposed to.*

What matters most for cognitive development

What helps babies pay attention, figure out patterns, and continue learning new things? In Chapters 1 and 2 we saw that sound sleep and less stimulation help baby's developing attention:

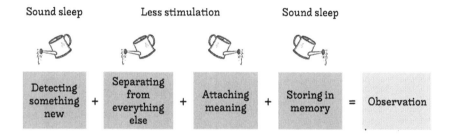

Sound sleep helps baby stay calm and regulated when he's awake so he can detect new things around him; when he goes to sleep again, his experiences are integrated into memory.[45, 46, 90] Less stimulation—less background noise, less unnatural movement, less visual clutter—helps baby separate new sounds, sensations, and sights from everything else and make sense of them.[9] Being rested and not overstimulated is especially important for young babies, but it continues to matter through the first year and beyond.

Babies accumulate their observations and figure out patterns naturally. It's easier for them to do so when they have opportunities to observe natural events in stable, predictable environments where they see the laws of physics and experience the patterns of human relationships again and again.

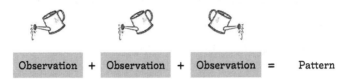

Stable, predictable environment

Observation + Observation + Observation = Pattern

For example, a baby may learn that when Mommy says "I'll be right back" and goes into another room, she's still nearby and always comes back in a few minutes; that a loud sound he sometimes hears comes from a family dog; that some toys float in a bathtub and others sink; that when food gets dropped, it falls down and he can no longer eat it; and when he looks at a book with Daddy, it will soon be time for bed. And eventually, babies learn to go back to sleep when they wake up and it's still dark—a very welcome pattern for their parents!

Finally, babies benefit from interacting with supportive adults and from exploring new objects safely and freely on their own:

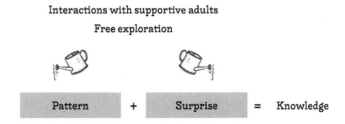

Interactions with supportive adults
Free exploration

Pattern + Surprise = Knowledge

Positive interactions help babies learn new actions and words, especially when adults actively support what babies are interested in. A study showed that when mothers routinely play with their babies in a positive but *less* stimulating way (allowing babies to lead and not tickling or excessively repositioning them), babies show neural activity indicative of stronger early brain development.[270] Exploring new things safely and freely on their own—for example, manipulating toys and play objects with different textures, weights, and shapes or simply watching natural events like a ray of sunlight travelling across the carpet—helps babies understand the world around them and develop mastery for more goal-directed play in later years.[276]

To summarize, this is what helps babies learn:

1. Sound sleep
2. Not too much stimulation
3. Seeing natural events in a stable, predictable environment
4. Interacting with supportive adults
5. Free exploration

Creating spaces for learning and development in our homes need not cost much, but it does require some careful thought and planning. We will explore some ways to do this in Part II.

Sensory and motor development

A newborn doesn't yet realize her own size, or that her hands and feet are connected to her. During the first year, as her sensory and motor development progresses, she will be mapping her own body and learning how to control it.

Sensory development refers to the perception and processing of information coming from various senses: touch, taste, smell, hearing, sight, balance, and proprioception (a sense of spatial orientation and movement). A very important component of sensory development is *sensory integration*: the ability of the brain to process and organize input received from multiple senses. Think of the various sensory inputs as pieces of a jigsaw puzzle: the brain has to put them together to form a complete picture. Science has shown that unlike most other aspects of development, sensitive windows for sensory integration occur very early in life.[274] Remember how pruning of the neural connections in the sensory cortex begins as early as eight months?[271] Early sensory experiences make a lifetime difference: by the time baby is eight months old, most of the neural connections in the sensory cortex have formed; some have strengthened and others remained weak based on what baby has experienced.

The fact that sensitive windows for sensory integration occur so early in life makes it important to identify and treat sensory problems, like eye misalignments and chronic ear infections, as early as possible. Babies can catch up later, but they may not be able to catch up fully if a sensory problem remains unnoticed for a long time.[274]

For sensory integration, babies need to engage multiple senses in a coordinated way: for example, they need to hear barking and see the dog at the same time. Unlike adults and older children, when babies look at something, they cannot simply shift their gaze to the side: they need to align their whole torso, head, and eyes and turn toward the object.[277] Because of this, babies benefit from being in positions that allow them to move safely and freely. Spending long periods of time in baby seats or swings limits a baby's visual field and thus reduces opportunities for sensory integration. So does watching events on a screen, which we will explore later in this chapter.

Motor development refers to baby's increasing ability to control her body movements; it includes gross motor skills like rolling over, sitting up, crawling, and walking, and fine motor skills like touching and manipulating objects. Motor development is very closely linked with sensory development: inputs from various senses determine which muscles are used, when, and how.

Scientific studies on babies' motor development used to largely focus on the timing of major milestones to create charts of "normal" development. Now scientists and practitioners agree that babies reach major milestones like sitting and walking in different ways and in their own time within broad ranges of typical development.[278] There is also less focus on *when* and more focus on *how* motor development unfolds to produce stability and mastery.

Motor development begins before birth and continues through natural, baby-initiated movement. Because babies sleep on their backs—the safest position for babies' sleep—the American Academy of Pediatrics recommends placing babies on their tummies when they're awake as much as possible:[111] a practice known as *tummy time*. Lifting up her head and eventually her upper body in this position strengthens a baby's neck and helps her practice extending actively against gravity. Such strengthening and antigravity extension are essential for developing stability in various weight-bearing positions such as being on hands-and-knees or sitting upright.[279]

Many parents struggle with tummy time because their babies seem to dislike it. Is it important then to place babies on their tummies? Several studies show that most healthy, full-term babies develop within normal range with or without tummy time; however, babies who do spend time on their tummies when awake tend to achieve developmental milestones earlier than babies who don't.[279] I haven't found any studies exploring how tummy time affects future quality of movement. I also haven't found any studies on tummy time for babies born prematurely or babies vulnerable to developmental delays; these babies may need more help in strengthening their muscles and developing coordination. It appears that, in general, tummy time is beneficial for motor development. In addition to (or instead of) the classic tummy time position—supervised, on a firm flat surface—baby can also spend time on her tummy lying on a parent's knees or chest. These positions also help strengthen the baby's neck and help her practice anti-gravity extension.

Babies benefit from natural movement in a variety of positions in which they are being safely supported.[279] When they feel comfortable, babies move their arms and legs freely, kick, wiggle, and eventually reach for things they are interested in. Most begin reaching for still objects between three and four and a half months, and for moving objects around four and a half months.[278] Moving their arms and legs, stretching, and reaching helps babies to naturally develop the strength and coordination they need for rolling over and sitting up. In fact, babies often roll over for the first time while trying to reach for something. This first roll usually surprises them, but by that point they've been getting ready for it for some time.

To sit up on their own, babies must develop core strength, upper body strength, and balance. Propping babies up with pillows and sitting them up in baby seats will not make them sit up independently faster. In fact, it may delay independent sitting, because these positions limit natural movement. Similarly, babies will not walk independently any sooner if they're held by their hands and "walked." Walking requires developmental readiness such as body proportions (babies' bodies catching up with their large heads), core and leg strength, and coordination. These developmental milestones cannot be taught. In a sense, babies mature, rather than learn, to walk. It happens when they're ready and when their environment allows for free movement.

There is another reason to not rush a baby into walking by helping her stay upright. Most (although not all) babies crawl before they walk. The crawling stage comes with a number of developmental benefits. Crawling helps strengthen the muscles and joints near the centre of the body—in baby's tummy, back, neck, hips, and shoulders—and helps develop postural control. As babies begin to crawl, they experiment with moving between different positions, like going from sitting to hands-and-knees and from hands-and-knees to sitting or standing, which requires shifting their weight, rotating, and bending. These transitional movements expand babies' freedom and independence, so they are not "stuck" sitting or standing. In addition to gross motor benefits, crawling helps with fine motor skills by developing arches, joints, and muscles in the hand.[280]

And, interestingly, crawling helps with brain development. A crawling baby's arms and legs move in opposition to one another. When a baby first begins crawling, he has to plan which arm goes first and which leg goes with it until crawling becomes automated and he no longer has to think about it. Such *motor planning* is believed to strengthen and coordinate neural activity.[281, 282] The same motor planning takes place when older children learn to jump, throw, or ride a bike. Refining and automating movements frees up children's brainpower for the thinking, reasoning, and creativity they need for formal learning.[283]

These findings do not mean that babies must be taught to crawl, which is not really possible anyway: some babies skip crawling and naturally progress straight to walking. What research points to is the benefits of giving babies the space and time to develop sensory and motor skills in their own, natural way.

Over the last number of years many models of baby play equipment have become available: swings, bouncy chairs, exer-saucer-type activity centres, baby jumpers, contoured pillows, moulded seats... the list goes on. Such devices keep babies stationary and have been aptly called "baby containers." Many come equipped with toys, and some with screens, for entertainment. Manufacturers often claim that such play equipment delivers developmental benefits. Yet research done so far has not found any. In fact, one study showed a correlation between time spent in "containers" and *slower* motor development, although all babies still developed within the typical range.[284] (This study did not include cases of very extensive use; if it had, it is plausible that not all babies would have followed the typical motor development progression.) Because "container" play equipment constrains natural movement by intent or by default, it is reasonable to expect that spending too much time in such equipment could delay motor development.

Two types of baby equipment are not recommended for use at any time. Baby walkers can cause injuries; they have been banned in Canada and discouraged from use in the United States. And some vibrating bouncy seats can get as loud as eighty-five decibels, which is far louder than a parent's voice.[248] Babies sitting in such seats would not be learning from being spoken to or from conversations happening around them.

The three developmental strands—social-emotional, cognitive, and sensory and motor—are tightly linked to one another. For example, motor development requires sensory integration and brain development. In turn, newly developed motor skills give babies fresh opportunities for learning as they expand their range of mobility and dexterity. They also allow babies to use familiar spaces and play materials in new ways.[278]

Play materials

Play is so vital for development that it has been a topic of quite a few scientific studies. The scientific definition of play is "an activity that is intrinsically motivated and results in joyful discovery."[285]

Many young animals play, including octopi, lizards, turtles, honey bees, rats, and monkeys. Play teaches young animals what they can and cannot do while they're protected from the pressures of adult life. For human babies, play also helps develop executive functioning of the brain, which is often described as self-regulation and planning. Executive functioning is important for many of the skills named most critical for the twenty-first century: creativity, problem solving, and collaboration.[285]

As babies grow, their play becomes more complex. Scientists categorize play into social categories (solitary, onlooker, parallel, and cooperative play) and cognitive categories (functional, constructive, and dramatic play).[286, 287] During the first year, babies mostly explore objects (functional play) and may begin manipulating them with a particular goal in mind (constructive play).

Scientific studies used to largely focus on the timing of when certain categories of play emerge, in order to create typical development charts. Now scientists and practitioners agree that babies' play does not progress linearly and that play categories alone should not be used to judge maturity. Well-rounded play environments include materials that encourage all types of play.[286]

As we learned earlier in this chapter, seeing natural events in a stable, predictable environment helps babies' cognitive development. Babies also benefit from exploring and manipulating safe, simple objects of different shapes, textures, and weights. These objects can be baby toys or safe household items like wooden bowls and spoons.

Because baby's mind and body are developing, she will not easily get bored: spaces and toys of yesterday offer new opportunities today. Play objects take on new meaning once a baby can manipulate them; different surfaces—a smooth wooden floor, a soft carpet, or tall grass—offer new possibilities for movement once a baby becomes mobile.[288] Babies are self-motivated explorers: during one hour of free exploration, new walkers average 2,400 steps, travel the distance of eight American football fields, and visit most of the available area and surfaces![289]

Do baby boys and girls need different toys? Several studies have shown that babies do seem to prefer stereotypical toys of their gender from an early age. When shown dolls and trucks, three- to eight-month-old girls look more at dolls and boys look more at trucks.[290] Older babies who are able to choose certain toys show similar preferences: boys play with cars and balls more, whereas girls tend to choose dolls and play food.[291] Preferences for types of toys *could* be innate, but it is also possible that adults consciously or subconsciously support stereotypical play by offering babies certain types of toys from the start.

And there's one activity that seems to fascinate girls and boys alike: watching screens.

Babies and screens

Today's homes have many screens: televisions, computers, tablets, and smart phones. When is a good time for babies to begin using them? This can be a topic of hot debate in parenting circles. Some families opt for a screen-free home altogether. Others believe screens should be introduced early. I recall a friend of mine, who was expecting her first baby at the time, remark, "Technology is essential nowadays; I will teach my son how to use educational apps as early as possible to set him up for success." Most families are somewhere in the middle.

In the 1970s, most children began watching television regularly around four years old.[292] Then, in the 1990s, baby-directed videos and television programs like the *Baby Einstein* series and *Teletubbies* began to appear. Most were marketed as educational tools that promoted brain development and cognitive skills. And by the early 2000s, the average age children began watching television became four *months* old. At three months, 40 percent of babies were already regular viewers; by two years, almost all babies were.[292] In 2005, every fifth child under two years old in the United States had a television set in their bedroom.[293]

> *Five-month-old Rylee is watching a television show. She is sitting very still and appears to be watching the screen intently.*
>
> Rylee can hear the sounds and see what's happening on screen almost as well as her big brother and her parents. She can recognize simple shapes. But all she's experiencing is a stream of flashing lights and colours with no apparent connection to each other, to the sounds she hears, or to the people and objects in her life. Rylee will not begin comprehending the show's content or even sequences of events until she is at least eighteen months old.[294, 295]

In a large survey completed in 2006, parents shared their reasons for letting babies and young toddlers watch television, DVDs, or videos. Most believed the programs were educational and good for their child's developing brain, and that viewing was enjoyable and relaxing.[292] Unfortunately, neither is true. Researchers have been actively looking into the effects of television and video exposure on babies and young children since the early 1990s, and at this point science has given us clear answers. Let's take a look at the television equation.

Negative effects

There are two negatives that are correlated with—and may be directly caused by—watching television. The first one is disrupted sleep. Babies who watch television tend to have less regular sleep[296] and generally sleep less.[123] Although the sleep loss is usually small, from a few minutes to half an hour per day, researchers warn that it can add up over time and create patterns that lead to a significant sleep deficit as the child grows.[123] Television viewing disrupts sleep in at least two ways. The blue light emitted from screens disrupts the production of melatonin, a hormone essential for healthy sleep.[297] In addition, viewing screens in itself is known to stimulate alertness.[293]

The second negative of watching television is overstimulation—and the effects it has on babies' developing attention. Rapid changes trigger babies' *orienting response*: a reflex that fixes their attention on new sights and sounds. This response is good and necessary; remember how babies learn from patterns and surprises? However, rapid-fire changes on screens are dizzying compared to the pace of real life—the pace the human brain spent millennia adapting to. Flashing lights and quick changes on screen overstimulate a baby's developing brain[294] as the part responsible for the orienting response fires away ("Alert! Change!"). This is why baby Rylee in our example above is sitting very still and watching intently. Her brain is trying to figure out what's happening ("Is this threatening? Is this important?"), but doesn't get the chance to process any input. Watching television is not relaxing for babies. In fact, it's likely stressful and exhausting!

As babies grow, their attention gradually develops from the orienting response toward *executive attention*, otherwise known as focus: they begin selecting specific information from sensory input.[298] Researchers believe that excessive television viewing may disrupt this natural process of attention development. The pacing of television shows, even those designed for babies, is extremely rapid compared with reality. Sensory overstimulation may condition children's developing brains to expect this level of stimulation and intensity in everyday lives. Some studies have found an association between very early exposure to television and attention problems. Children who watched two hours of television a day before age three had a 20 percent greater chance of attention problems in elementary school, compared to those who did not watch television as babies and toddlers; watching faster-paced shows was more strongly associated with subsequent attention problems.[299]

It is important to note that these studies found a correlation between screen time and attention—not causation. In other words, we cannot confidently conclude that screen time, or screen time alone, is the reason for later attention problems. To arrive at robust conclusions, one would need to conduct experiments that are not possible for ethical reasons. Thankfully, no researcher would purposefully expose young children to what is likely to be detrimental sensory overstimulation to see whether it would cause hyperactivity or cognitive impairment. So all studies on television viewing and attention in children have been—and will be—observational rather than experimental. Recently, however, an experiment was conducted on mice. Some young mice received excessive sensory stimulation: bright lights and sounds for six hours per day for six weeks (simulating a television-heavy household). These mice showed signs of impaired learning, impaired memory, increased risk-taking, and hyperactivity which researchers described as "ADHD-like."[268] We cannot directly extrapolate these findings to young humans, but they are important to consider as we may never have much more definitive answers from science.

There are several other negatives. They are not directly caused by television, but stem from what babies are *not* doing or getting during the time they are immersed in screens.

- Less interaction: Time babies spend watching screens is not spent interacting with caring adults or other children.
- Less free movement: During screen time babies are physically passive, often strapped in infant seats.
- Less learning: Remember how early babies can begin to grasp the laws of physics by recognizing patterns in daily life? The television world, however, does not have the same laws. In real life, a ball moving to the right will continue to move to the right until it stops. In contrast, a ball on screen moving to the right may disappear from view, only to reappear on the left to continue the rightward motion in an edited action sequence.[295] Watching screens does not help babies learn about the world around them.
- Less sensory integration: Sensory input coming from the screen is not as coordinated as real life.[300] For example, watching a flower on screen does not allow a baby to experience the full sensations of touching and smelling a real flower. Learning is harder without a complete picture.

These are, essentially, lost opportunities. Are they significant? They can be, depending on how much time babies spend watching. According to a large survey, three-month-olds on average watch about an hour each day.[292] This might not seem like much. But babies of this age sleep for sixteen or more hours per day and spend another three or so hours feeding and being changed and dressed. That means that screen time takes up almost a quarter of their awake time: a considerable portion. Remember how quickly brains are developing in the early years? Being in a screen-free environment gives babies more opportunities for connecting, building strength, exploring, and learning.

> ### Background Television
>
> In some families—approximately 40 percent in the United States—a TV is on all day, whether someone is watching or not.[301, 302] Background television still affects babies even when they're not actively watching the screen: it distracts them from interactions with their parents, they tend to play less, and their attention is less focused.[294, 303]

Positive effects

So what about the educational benefits claimed by the producers? The problem is, even if a show's content can be considered educational, babies are not developmentally ready to understand it. Watching screens is a demanding cognitive activity, one that requires special forms of attention, perception, and comprehension.[295] Babies develop these skills through exploring, connecting, and playing in the real world, not by watching screens.

Some videos claim to teach babies languages. The *Baby Einstein* series was inspired by the finding that young babies are sensitive to phonetic contrasts of any language, but at around six to nine months they begin to gradually lose this generalist sensitivity: their brains focus on the language they hear most. So *Baby Einstein* videos exposed babies to the sounds of many languages and were supposed to help them remain sensitive to many phonetic contrasts, to facilitate later language learning. However, videos like *Baby Einstein* don't work because babies learn best from live, human teachers. You might remember from Chapter 1 that newborns come ready to connect and learn from social interactions: they can recognize faces and voices and are sensitive to social cues like eye contact and facial expressions. A number of studies have now shown that babies learn much better from real people and real-life events than video—and that this "video deficit" phenomenon holds true until the child is two to three years old, and likely beyond.[294, 295, 304] In 2009, Disney offered refunds on *Baby Einstein* videos because its claims of learning benefits were unsupported. That being said, a plethora of "educational" videos and apps for babies have been developed since.

Some media content producers claim that their goal is to promote child-parent interaction. However, studies show that most parents do not watch television with their babies or toddlers.[292] Even when babies and their parents are watching together, they are probably interacting less than if they played with blocks, looked at a book, or even went about their daily activities together.

Overall, statements by television and video producers that their products are beneficial for babies are not supported by evidence. Most or all television and video content should not be marketed as educational or even developmentally appropriate for babies and toddlers. Yet there still appears to be a lack of regulation regarding such marketing claims.[300]

The effects of television on babies

Negative effects
- Disrupted sleep
- Overstimulation
- Potential risk to attention development
- Less interaction
- Less free movement
- Less learning
- Less sensory integration

Positive effects

None

What about mobile electronic devices like tablets and smart-phones? Many babies use their parents' devices and may even have their own, made specifically for young children. The effects of mobile technology are not yet well studied, but the list of neg-atives described above likely applies. Babies under one year old are exposed to the same type of content they would have been watching on television, but now from a mobile electronic device.

Moreover, some of the negatives may be amplified. Electronic devices are portable; many attach to car seats and strollers, lend-ing themselves as "electronic babysitters" to keep babies occu-pied during daily routines. This has the potential to increase babies' screen time in a very real but not easily noticeable way. In addition, mobile screens are smaller and positioned much closer to babies than television screens. This could have an even larger impact on babies' sleep because the blue light is stronger at close distances. Looking at screens up close for considerable amounts of time may also pose risks for babies' developing vision.[300] It may re-wire their visual systems toward up-close central fixation and lead to under-developed peripheral and distance vision.[305] The degree of these risks is currently unknown.

In summary, the one key consideration missing in the "babies and screens" debate is babies' development. Technology changes rapidly, but the needs of babies and young children—the biology of early childhood development—remain the same. Remember the five things that babies need for brain development: sound sleep, avoiding overstimulation, predictable environment, inter-actions with supportive adults, and free exploration? Of these five needs, screen time provides none.

Babies in daycare

Many babies transition to daycare as their parents return to work outside the home. This transition may happen when babies are a few weeks old or when they are closer to twelve months or older, depending on parental leave policies and family choices and circumstances.

The involvement of multiple adults in raising young children is not new or rare. For example, sharing baby-care responsibilities among several adults and older children is common in many African cultures.[306] In Western societies, some families have relatives who care for babies during their parents' absence, but most babies of working parents are cared for in group daycares by professional daytime caregivers.[307]

Unlike relatives, professional caregivers at a new daycare are new to the baby, and the daycare environment is often very different from home. This creates a big change in baby's world. On the plus side, parents are able to choose the type of daycare they prefer for their baby, a choice they would not have had if care were provided by relatives or friends. Perhaps because of this, parents want to see more research on daycare.[308] But studying daycare effects is not easy. True experiments are not possible, again for ethical reasons: researchers can't ask a group of parents, chosen at random, to send their babies to particular kinds of daycare. And in the absence of experiments it is difficult to determine cause and effect. But let's see what science can tell us despite these constraints.

Daycare attendance in itself does not disrupt child development

In the 1990s, a comprehensive and detailed study looked at associations between daycare and developmental outcomes by following a large, diverse group of over a thousand families in the

United States across their babies' first year and beyond.[309] This study showed that babies' attachment to their mothers was unrelated to the type, amount, or quality of daycare they attended, or the age the baby started attending daycare at. In other words, daycare in itself was neither a risk nor a benefit for the development of the baby-parent relationships. What mattered most for attachment—just as we saw earlier in this chapter—was parents' sensitivity. But when low parent sensitivity was combined with low-quality daycare, longer hours in daycare, or more than one daycare arrangement, the risks to the parent-baby relationship grew: in those cases, poor daycare experiences compounded the effects of insensitive home environments.[309]

Children in this study were subsequently followed into their preschool and elementary school years. In preschool, children who spent more than forty-five hours per week in daycare showed more behavioural problems than those who didn't.[310] Given how much babies and toddlers sleep, these children would have spent far more of their waking hours at daycare than at home. By Grade 5, more time spent in centre-based daycare in the early months and years was still associated with more behavioural problems.[311] However, parenting remained a stronger and more consistent predictor of development.[311]

Daycare environment is stressful for babies

Babies cannot tell us whether they are coping with stress, but researchers find out by measuring cortisol—a stress hormone—in babies' saliva. Across multiple studies, babies had higher cortisol concentrations on daycare days than on home days.[310, 312, 313] One study tracked cortisol levels during babies' first nine months at daycare. Cortisol levels were highest during the first month after transition, went down afterward, but nonetheless remained elevated compared to home days throughout the whole study period. This suggests that the daycare environment continued to be stressful for babies months after the transition. It is important to note, however, that elevated cortisol does not necessarily signal harm; elevated cortisol is an adaptive physiological response that shows a person is *experiencing* stress, and may or may not be *negatively affected* by it.

Although the ability to regulate emotions increases throughout the first year, babies go through many cognitive and motor milestones. These milestones bring challenges and novelty to cope with, which may be harder in a daycare setting.[312]

Interestingly, babies of sensitive parents tend to have a harder time adjusting to daycare, likely because of the greater contrast between their home environment and the less predictable and less personal daycare environment.[312, 314] Of course, this is not a call to be less sensitive at home. Quite the contrary: continuing to be a sensitive parent ultimately helps babies navigate their transition into daycare. What also helps is sound nighttime sleep. Babies and toddlers who sleep soundly have lower cortisol at daycare compared to babies and toddlers who do not sleep well at home.[315]

What about the quality of the daycare: does it help lower stress levels? Core features of high-quality daycares are safe and healthy spaces, developmentally appropriate stimulation, positive interactions with caregivers, and a focus on the individual child's emotional growth.[316] Researchers assess these features by observing children and caregivers during the daycare's daily routines. Studies show that daycare quality does matter for toddlers and preschoolers: across different nations, children in lower-quality daycares have higher cortisol levels compared to children in higher-quality daycares.[317] However, the effects of daycare quality have not yet been comprehensively studied for babies under one year old. What we do know is that babies form relationships with their caregivers—and that these relationships are important.

Who the caregivers are and what they do matters

A caregiver can become baby's attachment figure, and the type of attachment to a caregiver can differ from baby's attachment to her parents. In other words, it is possible for a baby to have a secure attachment to her caregiver even if she doesn't have secure attachments at home, and the other way around. Not surprisingly, babies benefit most when all of the attachment relationships in their lives—to family members and to any other caregivers—are stable and secure.[318]

However, not all caregivers value sensitive caregiving and support attachment: across studies in multiple countries, warm and supportive relationships between babies and their caregivers were generally seen less than half of the time.[316, 319] Some caregivers avoid attachment to encourage babies' independence. Other caregivers believe that attachment conflicts with professionalism, and yet others are concerned that parents would resent them should babies become attached to them.[320] Fortunately, there are caregivers who value and foster attachment and "professional love"[321]—the deep connection that emerges through being with babies and seeing them as individual beings with unique needs. For these caregivers, loving babies in their care is a core element of their professional identity.[322] Their professional love does not seek to compete with the love between babies and their parents, but rather complements it.[321]

In some daycare centres, all caregivers take turns caring for all babies. Other centres use the **primary caregiver model** where one caregiver consistently tends to a group of babies. Research supports the primary caregiver model, showing that stability of care and time spent together help develop attachment.[323, 324] This model allows caregivers to get to know the babies in their care well, and babies to learn to trust the knowledgeable, understanding, and consistent adult—their key person at daycare.

> *The best daycares for babies have sensitive, tuned-in staff, practise the primary caregiver model, and provide dedicated and safe spaces to rest, eat, move, and explore.*

Babies are most at ease at daycares where caregivers' interaction styles are similar to what they experience at home with their parents.[306] Recognizing familiar interaction patterns and, eventually, words helps babies feel more secure. In addition, trusting relationships between parents and daycare staff develop faster when there is a close match between the family's values and the values and vision of the daycare centre.[325] However, parents' options are usually limited by daycare location, hours, cost, or space availability. As a result, caregiver beliefs around control and support—for example, whether emotional expression is to be encouraged and whether verbal reprimands and punishments are acceptable—are often very different from those of babies' parents. These discrepancies tend to prevail over time, even if the communication between caregivers and parents improves.[306] This highlights the importance of choosing, from the start, a daycare centre that is a good fit for the baby.

Overall daycare environment matters more than specific activities

"Curriculum" and "educational programming" are increasingly used in descriptions of infant and toddler daycares. This could be a good thing, as long as the focus is on careful planning of the environment and experiences, and not on school readiness.[326] The best learning environments for babies are those that are restful and nurturing. Indirect lighting, noise control, and dedicated, quiet spaces for sleep and rest are important for babies' development.[9] Babies also need safe spaces to move and explore. In daycare centres babies spend a significant portion of their awake time indoors, often in the meals area in seats and high chairs.[327] Daycare centres that recognize the value of free movement and exploration provide stimulating and safe spaces for babies to move, both indoors and outdoors.

INFANT DEVELOPMENT: KEY POINTS

- Babies sense their parents' support and learn to anticipate it at only a few weeks old. A close, committed relationship with at least one adult is crucial for their social-emotional development. Close relationships form best when parents are sensitive and mind-minded.
- Babies learn through paying attention: observing, figuring out patterns, and noticing surprising events. Getting sound sleep, receiving less stimulation, observing natural events in stable, predictable environments, interacting with supportive adults, and exploring freely help cognitive development.
- Natural, baby-initiated movement is important for sensory integration and motor development.
- Early relationships are central to all aspects of development: social-emotional, cognitive, sensory, and motor.
- Watching television and other screens does not benefit any aspects of development and may cause negative effects.
- Daycare attendance in itself does not disrupt child development or parent-baby relationships, but the choice of daycare matters.

Let's explore what we can do to create the best environments for connecting, growing, and learning.

PART II
AN ENVIRONMENT FOR CARE AND PLAY

"Caring for children is not a kind of work… but a kind of love"
—Dr. Alison Gopnik,
The Gardener and the Carpenter

A few decades ago, many parents believed that babies who were responded to quickly and held a lot would grow into ungrateful, manipulative, spoiled children.[328] Fortunately, we now know enough about child development to be confident that our attention does not "spoil" babies. Babies never manipulate us, but simply communicate their needs and feelings. Our sensitive and mind-minded responses are vital for babies' development: they strengthen attachment, help babies develop trust, allow them to learn, and help them regulate emotions during babyhood and beyond.

This could have surprised your grandparents back in the day, but I bet it doesn't surprise you or most young parents you know, which is wonderful. Yet, as society learns more about early childhood development, another narrative is beginning to emerge: that we must take advantage of the early windows of opportunity and enhance our babies' development before it's too late. In addition to the "protected" vision of childhood that focuses on the child's well-being in the moment, the "prepared" vision concentrates largely on the future: preparing children for success in adult life.[329] This "prepared" vision has inspired a multitude of educational toys and baby-enrichment classes. Electronic toys and apps immerse babies in music and foreign languages; flashcards provide stimulation; lessons such as "multi-sport class for babies as young as four months" and "infant aquatics" are available. Do these toys and activities truly prepare our babies for a better future?

Looking closely at the science of infant development has made it clear to me: during the early months and years, protecting *is* preparing. By sensitively and mindfully protecting our babies from overtiredness, too much stimulation, and too fast of a pace, we give them more opportunities to experience our love and care, to play and explore freely, to figure out how the world works through the patterns of everyday life, and to discover themselves. This allows for the natural, gradual development of their identity, well-being, creativity, and strength.

Protecting our babies from overtiredness and overstimulation nurtures their well-being in the moment and prepares them for the future.

I now invite you to think about the science of child development as you create the environment for your baby's care and play. The three building blocks are: (1) safe, simple spaces, (2) connection through care and play, and (3) free movement and exploring:

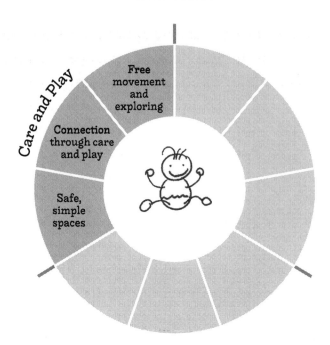

The ONE approach: Universal building blocks for care and play.

There are many ways to create environments that are safe, nurturing, and conducive to learning. As you prepare to create yours, ask yourself the following questions. There are no right or wrong answers, and your answers may change later on. Answer as you see things today.

- How will I adapt my home once my baby is here? Once she becomes mobile?
- What are my thoughts around toys? Would I like my baby to have a small selection or a large variety of toys?
- What do I want my baby to learn about interactions between people in our family?
- Would I want my baby to spend a considerable amount of time on his own, with a caring adult nearby but without active interaction? Why or why not?
- What does play mean to me?
- How do I want my baby to feel about her body as she grows?

- What are my thoughts around babies doing things that are hard for them (for example, waiting to be fed; struggling to roll over; feeling frustrated when playing)? What, if any, challenges do I consider to be good for my baby? At what age?
- Do I want my baby to participate in educational activities outside our home?
- Besides our immediate family, who do I want my baby to form relationships with?

Keep your vision in mind as you put the first building block in place: safe, simple spaces for care and play.

Safe, simple spaces

Some parents completely rearrange their home to prepare for baby's arrival. Good friends of ours turned their living room into a playroom and fully baby-proofed the rest of the house as soon as they found out their baby was on the way. Other families prefer fitting baby things into their adult-oriented home. Whichever approach you choose, think about arranging your home in a way that will work for your whole family. Baby care and play spaces do not need to be extensive or expensive, but they must be set up carefully and thoughtfully. These spaces work best when they're simple, comfortable, and convenient for you and safe, familiar, and engaging for your baby. We already talked about sleep and feeding spaces in Chapters 2 and 3. Let's now think about spaces for diapering, bathing, and play.

Spaces for diapering and bathing

Depending on your home's layout, you may want to set up one dedicated diaper changing area or make multiple changing stations. Most babies need a middle-of-the-night diaper change for at least the first couple of months. Set up a diaper changing area next to where your baby sleeps, so you don't have to carry her into another room in the middle of the night. Arrange all the supplies—diapers, wipes, receiving blankets, and a couple changes of clothes—within arm's reach. This is especially important if you're using a changing table or a mat placed on a dresser or bed. Never take your hands off your baby when she's on an elevated surface, even for a second, even if she's never rolled over before: you never know when she'll do it for the first time. I found it easier and safer to change my babies on a waterproof mat on the floor starting at around six weeks (when I was physically able to get down to the floor and up again comfortably and safely); that way I was sure they wouldn't fall.

Your baby's changing table may come with a hanging mobile or toys, but these are not necessary. In fact, not having distractions around the changing area might help you in the long run… or more accurately, in the wiggle-and-crawl-away stage. Many babies begin resisting diaper changes as they gain mobility: they wiggle, flip over, and try to crawl or walk away. Common advice for this stage is to ride it out by letting your baby be on all fours or standing up as you change him, but in reality that's hard to do without making a mess. Instead, try to connect with your baby and involve him in each diaper change from the early days, so he feels like an active participant.

Bathing will become part of your baby's rhythm early on. You don't necessarily need a special baby bath: some parents like to use the sink or the adult bathtub. In either case it's important to place all of your bathing supplies—soap, wash cloth, towel, and a fresh diaper and clothes—within arm's reach because you should never turn away from your baby when he's in the bath. Always check the water temperature before you lower your baby in; I found a bath thermometer helpful as my ability to correctly judge water temperature seems to depend on how warm or cold I feel myself. I also liked having an inclined mesh bath sling for bathing my babies: it seemed to help them feel more comfortable and secure in the water.

Now that you've planned dedicated areas for diapering and bathing, think about making the rest of your home baby-friendly.

A baby-friendly home

When your baby becomes mobile, you'll want to make sure your home is safe for him to navigate: place safety gates around staircases and fireplaces, cover electrical outlets, remove all chemicals and choking hazards from baby's reach, secure any loose cords and unstable furniture, and make other adjustments. Crawl around your home to see it from your baby's vantage point to discover hidden dangers and trouble spots you might not have thought about. You will easily find detailed checklists and specialized products for baby-proofing online.

But there's one aspect of making your home baby-friendly that's not frequently discussed, and it's one you might want to think about before your baby becomes mobile, and even before he's born. We saw in Part I that a simple, calm atmosphere helps babies develop self-regulation and attention, which are important for social-emotional development and learning. One of the best ways to bring in more simplicity and calm to your home is to slow down and reduce noise by limiting background television and overall screen use.

Practical Tips for Reducing Noise
and Screen Time in Your Home:

Save your own screen time for when your baby is sleeping. This
advice may seem obvious, but it's surprisingly easy to get into the
habit of using television, a tablet, or a phone during the long feedings in the early weeks and months. Try to avoid screens when you
feed your baby, especially at nighttime when stimulation and blue
light can interfere with sleep.

Limiting screen time can be challenging if you or your family
members are used to having the television on in the background. If
you want to turn television off and find alternative ways to "occupy
the house," try playing soft music or listening to podcasts some of
the time.

We learned in Part I that screen time is associated with disrupted sleep and sensory overstimulation in babies, which in
turn correlates with attention deficits later in childhood. We will
likely never know whether screen time, or screen time alone,
causes later attention problems because controlled experiments
needed to answer this question conclusively would be unethical. Yet, in a sense, our society is already engaged in a large and
uncontrolled experiment where many babies and toddlers grow
up immersed in electronic media. The technology we embrace
as a family becomes normal for our children. We have control
over media's place in our homes and in our young children's daily
lives. I believe the knowledge we currently have—the negative
effects of screen time on attention discovered in animal studies,
as well as correlations found in human babies—are important to
consider as we make decisions for our families.

The American Academy of Pediatrics (AAP) recommended
no television viewing for children younger than two years old

in 1999. This recommendation was reiterated and extended to mobile technology in 2011. In 2016, the AAP issued an update recommending no screen time except for video-chatting for children under eighteen months, and carefully chosen high-quality programming, watched with a parent, beyond eighteen months. In 2019 the World Health Organization recommended no screen time for children under two years old.

Major health guidelines recommend no screen time during baby's first year and beyond.

These guidelines are well aligned with scientific research. However, many parents don't follow them: for example, in the early 2000s almost every second baby in the United States was watching television regularly by three months old.[292] Many families don't follow screen time recommendations now, and you can probably guess why. As mentioned earlier, parents allow their babies to have screen time because they believe it's good for their child's developing brain, enjoyable, and relaxing (none of which is true, according to science). But another common reason is that parents need time to get things done.[292] This is an important and valid reason. You may be working from home, taking care of older children or other family members, or recovering from an illness while taking care of your baby. And no doubt sometimes you simply need time for yourself.

Discussions on screen time in early childhood all too often turn to parent-shaming and don't offer any alternatives. But alternatives do exist, including those that give you an opportunity to get things done or take a break. The answer, once again, lies in the types of activities that help babies learn: sleep, free exploration, and interactions with supportive adults. We already talked about developing sleep rhythms and routines in Chapter 2. One of the easiest ways to help your baby explore freely is to create a dedicated, one hundred percent safe space for play in your home.

A safe play area

Consider creating a special enclosed area in your home for your baby to explore and play in. This could be a play yard, a gated-off area or a whole room if your home allows. The most important thing is that this play area must be absolutely, completely safe for your baby. It cannot be *almost* completely safe: "I just have to watch that he doesn't pull on the blinds" means the area is *not* completely safe. Magda Gerber, the founder of the Resources for Infant Educarers, invited parents to think of a "safe place" as so safe that if you accidentally got locked out of the house, your baby might end up hungry and wet, but would be completely unharmed.[330] Of course, getting yourself locked out of the house is never recommended, but you get the idea.

In theory, a crib—an enclosed, safe, and simple space—fits the description of a safe play area. When I was a baby, my family lived in a tiny shared apartment, and my crib doubled as my play area. However, I recommend making your baby's play area separate from her sleeping space if possible. It'll be easier for your baby to develop sustainable sleep associations when her sleeping space is used for sleep only. Also, as you know, there should be no toys in your baby's sleeping space for safety reasons. If you keep sleep and play spaces separate, you won't need to worry about removing toys before your baby goes to sleep.

One simple way to create a play area is to enclose part of a room using safety gates. Gates may seem confining to adults, but to babies they can provide a sense of safety and freedom. As your baby figures out routines and patterns and becomes used to his play area, he will know that he's free to explore. He won't bump his head on a sharp corner or keep hearing "no" as he probably does when he navigates other spaces set up for adults or older children. In her book *Elevating Childcare*, Janet Lansbury calls safe play areas "yes spaces" for just that reason.[331]

A play area can be set up very simply: a flat surface to move on freely and a few safe play objects. Babies who aren't yet mobile or are learning to roll will be most comfortable on a mat or a carpet; babies who crawl can benefit from having a carpeted area and a slippery floor to scoot or slide on, if your space allows for both. You don't need any special decorations: the natural sights and sounds in your home will be enough. Even school-age children whose attention is more developed still get distracted in environments with bright, busy decorations.[332]

The biggest benefit of a designated play area is that it allows your baby to experiment safely and to focus on his interests uninterrupted. For example, a nine-month-old pulling everything off a shelf might be exploring how different objects fall. This could be a problem in the living room, but a great activity in a safe play area where the shelf is low and secure and play objects are soft, light, and unbreakable. A safe play area offers your baby what early childhood educators call "scaffolding": just the right help, at just the right time, in just the right way to support development and learning. You can give your baby just the right support—an interesting environment, complete safety, and uninterrupted time—so she can focus on what interests her most. She is free to explore, learn, and master new tasks at her own pace.

You might wonder whether having one consistent play area would eventually become boring for your baby. But remember how quickly her cognitive and motor development progresses. As her new skills emerge, they enrich and expand her play environment naturally.[278] She won't easily get bored of the same space because she will continue to discover new ways to use it. For example, in the early months she might be interested in gazing at the light coming from the window; later on she'll begin pulling up and perhaps cruising while holding on to the window sill; later yet, she might begin to purposefully arrange her toys along the edge. You can introduce new play objects as you notice your baby's skills and interests grow. When you add play objects, and every time your baby masters a new skill, re-assess her play area: is it still completely safe?

Last but not least, a safe play area will be helpful for you, particularly if you have older children or pets, or work from home. It separates baby's space and allows you to go to the bathroom or answer the phone without worry—and without having to bring your baby with you every time, holding her or placing her in a seat or swing.

What a Safe Play Area Provides

- An opportunity for your baby to move freely and explore uninterrupted
- A consistent but interesting environment for your baby
- Peace of mind for you when you need to step away or have your hands free

---

Toys and play objects: a stage-by-stage guide

"I'd rather see a busy child actively manipulating a simple toy in a variety of creative ways ... than see a passive child playing with a busy toy" — Magda Gerber,
Your Self-Confident Baby

Your baby's play objects can include store-bought or handmade toys as well as household items you already have on hand: anything that is safe for your baby to explore by handling and mouthing. Here are a few ideas on how to choose play objects for your baby.

✓ **All play objects must be safe and easy to clean**. As a rule of thumb, all play objects must be large enough to not fall through a toilet paper roll. They must not come apart into small pieces that a baby could choke on, and must be free of strings or sharp edges. The materials should be safe for a baby to mouth; cloth, silicone, natural rubber, unpainted wood, and phthalate-free plastic are good options. Toys must also be easy to clean: avoid materials that are not washable. Finally, watch for toys that can trap water or a baby's saliva inside and get mouldy, a common problem with rubber duckies and other bath toys, teethers, and toys with squeakers. Look for toys that are fully sealed.

✓ **Good play objects follow the laws of physics.** The best "learning toys" aren't necessarily marketed as such, and often don't have many bells and whistles. Simpler toys are better at helping babies learn how the world works. Your baby will enjoy exploring various textures, shapes, weights, densities, and colours. If you want to introduce toys and objects that make noise, choose ones that allow your baby to understand *how* the noise is made. For example, as your baby plays with a toy drum or a spoon and a plastic container, she will learn that banging objects together makes a sound. She will also learn that the sound varies depending on how soft the object is and how hard she hits it, and that hitting water makes a splash; she will be using all her senses. If she's curious about sounds, she'll keep experimenting, which will advance her strength, fine motor skills, and sensory integration, and give her a sense of mastery. She won't learn any of that from simply pressing a button on an activity table or swiping a touchscreen on a smart-phone. Yes, electronic toys and devices teach her how to press and swipe. But if you think about it, these tasks are very simple, can be learned any time in life, and are rather meaningless on their own. To use electronic devices in a meaningful way, one must first understand how the real world works outside of the screen.

✓ **Great play objects can be used in a variety of ways.** Older babies benefit from exploring toys they can do multiple things with. For example, a small bucket can be filled and emptied, held to the face and spoken into, turned upside down to stack objects on, swung from side to side, and carried from place to place. Open-ended toys like this help babies naturally transition from simply manipulating objects to constructive play: doing something with a partic-ular goal in mind.[333] Unlike mechanical and electronic toys, these simple toys do nothing on their own, and this leaves more possibilities for your baby to come up with different ways to use them.

When is a good time to introduce play objects? A newborn doesn't yet need toys: the sites and sounds around him are enough to stimulate his senses. A very young baby may be con-tent just looking around or exploring his hands or pyjama sleeves. Introduce play objects when you notice your baby is beginning to actively reach for and grab objects. This usually happens at around three months.

Safe, Open-Ended Toys and Play
Objects: Ideas for Various Stages

3–6 months: wooden and silicone rings and other simple, easy-to-hold shapes; cloth napkins of different textures; linkable plastic rings; crinkly toys; wooden spoons

6–9 months: silicone muffin cups; cloth and board books; simple musical instruments (shakers, bells, drums); cloth dolls and stuffed animals

9–12 months: nesting cups; stacking toys; balls (wiffle-type balls are easiest for baby to manipulate); toy buckets; sturdy plastic and wooden containers; simple cars; large blocks; hats; sturdy baskets and boxes.

Your baby will continue enjoying these simple toys well into his second year. He will find new ways to play with them as he masters new skills.

There is no need to choose gender-specific toys. Boys and girls will benefit from a variety of toys and play objects including cars and dolls.

If your baby is not yet mobile, you can simply place a few play objects within her reach. For an older baby you may want to arrange the toys on low open shelves or in baskets, a few toys in each so they are easy to see. Shelves and baskets will be easier for your baby to use than deep toy boxes and chests.

How many toys does a baby need? The average number of toys in a North American middle-class home is between 90 and 140—and that's not the total number, but the number researchers could see *at once* (standing in one spot) as they visited the families.[333] The United States represents 3.1 percent of the world's children, but 40 percent of the toy market.[333] But having too many choices may distract children and inhibit their creativity. For example, in one study toddlers were offered either sixteen or four toys; they played with the four toys for longer and in a greater variety of ways. Researchers believe that having fewer distractions gave these toddlers an opportunity to pay greater attention and encouraged them to explore the objects more deeply.[333]

We can begin simplifying the number and complexity of our children's toys when they're babies. If you want to offer your baby a large variety of toys, consider rotating them: having only some of the toys available at any given time. Small, manageable collections of toys can be played with while the majority is stored away. Watching your baby play will help you decide how many toys to offer at a time; you can then remove a few and add new ones every week or every couple of weeks. This approach will help bring novelty without the distraction of having too many toys available.[333] A small number of interesting toys and play objects in a safe area will create an interesting space for your baby to explore.

Let's now look at the second building block of the care and play environment: connection through care and play.

Connection through care and play

We saw earlier in this chapter that babies learn about the world much like scientists do: they carefully observe people and things around them, figure out patterns, and form expectations and theories. Some of these observations are about the physics and biology of their surroundings. Others are about people, relationships, and feelings, including respect, connection, and love.

In *The Philosophical Baby*, Dr. Alison Gopnik writes that when a child is forming a theory about the physical or biological world, she has a large and consistent data set: for example, most balls fall down rather than up; most seeds grow to be plants. But when it comes to love, the child has to draw conclusions based on a very small and variable sample: mom, dad, siblings, and close family and friends.[273] What we do and what our babies see matters greatly.

When you hear "quality time with your baby," what comes to mind? For many parents it's playtime: playing peekaboo or building a tower of blocks together. Play is, indeed, a wonderful opportunity for quality time, but so are day-to-day caregiving routines. You will be spending a lot of time taking care of your baby, with at least three thousand diaper changes and feedings in the first year. When done with full attention, these routines can be wonderful opportunities for quality time and connection.

Quality time = any time of emotional connection between a baby and a parent or caregiver.

Connected caregiving

Being with babies and responding to them with sensitivity and mind-mindedness gives babies emotional roots: trust in the people they love, a sense of self-worth and competence, and a growing understanding of their own emotions and the emotions of others. Remember that sensitivity means responding to your baby's needs not only promptly, but also adequately. A response is adequate when it is well-matched to your baby's needs, emotions, and developmental level, as well as to the particular situation you and your baby are in.[26]

You can practice connected caregiving by recognizing and anticipating your baby's needs, caring for her with respect, and figuring out the roots of any challenging behaviour before responding.

Recognizing and anticipating needs

You won't always know what your baby needs and what to do, and that's normal and perfectly okay. It will get easier as you get to know your baby, and as she grows. When your baby is crying and you don't know what she needs, move close or pick her up. Then, take a moment to pause and try to understand what your baby might be telling you. Don't immediately offer her a pacifier. Remember that crying is the only way she can communicate her needs, emotions, and states. Pausing may not be easy; it's difficult to hear your baby or child cry. We are biologically wired to "do something, do anything" as babies' crying immediately activates parts of our brains urging us to move and speak. But quite often a brief pause will help you figure out what your baby needs.

> *I was walking with two-month-old Tessa in the stroller when she suddenly began to cry hard. I thought she must be hungry; it was winter and we were both bundled up, so I decided to head home. As soon as we got home I tried to feed her, but she wasn't interested. She was still crying, and her cry had a different pitch to it. When I finally went to undress and change her, I discovered that a microfibre insert in her diaper had shifted upward and was irritating her sensitive skin. It took a while for the rash to heal—and for me to stop feeling upset that I didn't notice the problem sooner. I learned that day that when Tessa cried with that particular pitch, she was communicating physical discomfort.*

To make it easier for your baby to communicate his needs—and for you to understand him—protect your baby from overstimulation and overtiredness as much as you can. Less background noise, less unnatural movement, less visual clutter will help him separate his sensations and needs from everything else, begin to make sense of them, and communicate them to you. Sound sleep will help your baby stay calmer and more regulated when he's awake. To help your baby stay well-rested, remember to look for "soft" tiredness cues: the slight quieting, staring off, calmness, a lull in energy. Eye rubbing, fussiness, and crying are usually signs of an overtired baby.

Similarly, you don't need to wait for your baby to start crying to feed him: crying is a late hunger sign. Look for the early hunger clues: increased alertness, turning his head to one side in a rooting way, or opening his mouth. Follow your baby's rhythms as you establish—and then support—daily routines that make his life predictable and cozy.

Transitions to care routines

When you are ready to pick up your baby to feed him, change his diaper, or put him into a car seat, wait a few seconds until he's paying attention to you. If he's playing or exploring, don't interrupt: giving him a few moments to complete his observations encourages focus and attention. When he is ready, tell him what you're going to do. If your baby is older than five months, he will likely understand some of your words; if he's younger, he'll be learning them as he hears them day after day. Talk *to* your baby rather than *about* him. Telling your partner "I'll go feed Jack" will not be enough for your young baby to register your words or anticipate what comes next; remember, babies rely on eye contact and our body language to help them understand we are talking to them and process that communication. Make eye contact with your baby and use short, simple sentences.

Your older baby is unlikely to understand	Your older baby will likely understand
I'll go feed the baby.	I am going to pick you up to feed you.
Let's go splish-splash, okay?	It's bath time.

Move slowly and approach your baby in such a way that you're visible to him. Remember, even two-month-olds can anticipate being picked up and will adjust their posture accordingly. Your baby might look at your face, tense his neck and back muscles, and open his arms a little wider, creating space for your hands. This will make picking your baby up smoother and safer, and will also give him an opportunity to participate in a joint routine from a very young age. When you carry your baby, make sure he's fully supported against your body so he feels comfortable and safe.

Caring with respect

As you care for your baby, move slowly, talk to him, and respond to the sounds he makes, letting him know what you're about to do. As your baby grows, you can begin asking him to help. For example, during a diaper change he can hold a fresh diaper or cloth, lift his bum, or work on undoing a snap on a pyjama or putting his legs into pants. Soon your baby will recognize the patterns and begin to anticipate diaper changing as an activity *he does with you*, as opposed to something that has to be *done to him* multiple times each day.

Show your baby from the start that her body is to be treated respectfully and lovingly. Begin teaching her, early on, that all her body parts have names. Don't use negative language when referring to diaper contents, gas, or burping.

Instead of saying	Consider saying
Eww, your bum is stinky!	I am going to change your diaper.

Practice mind-mindedness by trying to understand how your baby is feeling and naming the expressions you see. This will help your baby learn about emotions, begin recognizing them, and have the words to express them later on.[259]

Instead of saying	Consider saying
You're okay!	You pinched your finger and it hurts. You are *upset*.
Someone sure is excited.	You are *hungry* for lunch today!
Don't cry, it's just a puppy.	You seem *scared* of the dog. I will ask if he is friendly and if I can pet him.

It is natural to want to comfort your baby when she's hurt or upset, but saying "You're okay" or "It's just a…" can be confusing. When children are upset they don't feel okay. Hearing "You're okay" may, in the long run, inadvertently teach a child to not trust her feelings or express them fully.

In the examples above it's not the exact words that matter; it's mind-mindedness that does. When you think about the situation from your baby's perspective and acknowledge his feelings, you'll find the words that fit best.

Challenging behaviour

All behaviour has meaning. Babies communicate to us what they're working on and what's hard for them. Challenging behaviour can usually be explained by one of three reasons: developmental stage, difficult conditions, and testing limits and boundaries. Whenever you find your baby's behaviour challenging, ask yourself the following questions:

Is this behaviour part and parcel of the developmental stage my baby's going through?

Reason for behaviour	Examples	Solutions
Developmental stage[334,335]	• a two-month-old with colic crying inconsolably • a four-month-old waking multiple times at night for two weeks in a row	Prioritize rest for your baby and yourself; adjust your expectations; take care of yourself; wait it out.

Is something in my baby's surroundings causing this behaviour?

Reason for behaviour	Examples	Solutions
Difficult conditions[334,335]	• a tired six-month-old fussing in a public place • an eight-month-old crying hard when held by someone she doesn't know • a ten-month-old wanting to touch and mouth everything on low shelves at a relative's house	Take your baby out of the situation if/when possible; acknowledge your baby's struggle and hold and comfort her through distress.

Is my baby beginning to test what she can and cannot do?

Reason for behaviour	Examples	Solutions
Testing limits and boundaries	• a ten-month-old persistently crawling toward the fireplace despite being told not to • a twelve-month-old throwing food on the floor	Baby-proof your home; create a completely safe play area for your baby to explore; begin setting boundaries of behaviour.

A good starting point is to consider your baby's developmental stage. Is your baby's behaviour something to be fully expected at this stage? Are you normally okay with it, but find it difficult today because you're tired or distracted? This might be a sign that you need rest or time for yourself.

Next, think about the situation or conditions you and your baby are in: what might be challenging for your baby, and what can you do to help? Much of what parents find difficult—for example, crying or fussing in places or situations that demand quiet—are babies' natural responses to tiredness or overwhelm. These are largely beyond your baby's control, but something *you* can help with by taking your baby out of the overwhelming situation or by comforting him. As you may recall from Part I, when babies' needs are met consistently, their nervous systems practice shifting between different states, and staying calm and returning to a calm state becomes easier for them.

Finally, think about whether your older baby might be starting to test limits or boundaries. Babies test their physical surroundings to learn about them from a very young age. They mouth objects to explore their properties; they take their socks and shoes off (and usually put them in their mouth); they drop, spill, open, and empty. When your baby becomes mobile, usually around nine months, he will begin testing limits of what *he* can physically do by climbing, reaching, and pulling. He will repeat his tests because he needs to verify the results: I couldn't climb on the step stool yesterday, but will I be able to do it today? The best way to address physical testing is to baby-proof your home, create a safe play area for your baby to explore freely, and watch him closely, especially when visiting an unfamiliar place. Create opportunities for your baby to explore the properties of different objects and his own abilities by offering safe choices: for example, toys to mouth and obstacles to practice climbing on and off, like gymnastics mats or couch cushions.

Your baby might also begin testing the boundaries of behaviour: figuring out what she can and cannot do, and how decisions are made in your family. Many children don't test boundaries of behaviour until toddlerhood, but some begin near the end of their first year. Twelve-month-olds are able to read the emotional expressions of their parents and change their own behaviour depending on how parents respond (remember the experiment with the plexiglass-covered drop-off?). For example, your baby might take off her bib and look at you quizzically: is this okay or will you put it back on, Mommy? Similar to how she tests the physical world, she will repeat testing again and again because she needs to verify her results: is something that was not allowed yesterday still not allowed today?

This type of testing can be challenging for parents. Here are several considerations to help you feel more confident and supported:

✓ Testing is healthy. It reflects your baby's growing cognitive and social skills.

✓ Testing is not manipulation. Your baby is not testing *you*, he is testing his own abilities. He is becoming aware that he can have an impact on his environment and on people around him. This is a powerful and important realization, one we must support by recognizing it and creating appropriate boundaries.

✓ Setting boundaries is not punishment. On the contrary, boundaries help children stay safe and comfortable: like guardrails, boundaries show children they are safe, that caring adults won't let them go too far. Boundaries keep a child's world to a size they can comfortably manage.[204]

When you set a boundary, use simple and direct statements ("I don't want you to pull my hair"). Your baby is likely to understand at least some of the words and will pick up on your intonation. Boundaries disguised as questions ("What are you doing?") will confuse him.

Instead of saying	Consider saying
Stop that, what are you doing, silly? We don't throw food. Can you stop, please?	I don't want you to throw food. It looks like you are done eating. I will clean you up.

Help your baby stop the behaviour gently but firmly. The more consistent you are from day to day, the easier it will be for your baby to recognize the patterns and to understand what you want her to do (or not do).

Many parents find early boundary-setting difficult or confusing. So far you have been responding to all of your baby's needs, and now it can be hard to say "no" to her. However, consider another way of looking at it: having consistent, clear boundaries now *is* one of your baby's needs. She's learning about safe and acceptable behaviour and other important lessons.

Twelve-month-old Frida pulls off her sunhat when playing in the backyard. Her mom says, "I want you to wear your hat. It protects you from the bright sun," and puts it back on. Frida takes it off again; the cycle repeats a few more times. Frida's mom says, "You need a hat when we are outside. I see you are having trouble keeping it on. I am going to take you in." Frida begins to cry. Her mom gently picks her up, carries her inside, and holds her through the tears. They will try again after lunch.

It will take a few more experiences like this for Frida to learn that she must wear a hat when playing outside in the sun. She is also learning that her mom follows through when she says no, and that her mom is there for her when she is upset. Ultimately, Frida is learning that all of her feelings are okay, but some actions are not.

Whenever you spend time figuring out the reason behind your baby's challenging behaviour, you practise skills you will need for many years to come. Try to go beyond simply stopping the behaviour; reflect on why it might be happening, how you can help your baby, and what you want to teach her. This approach will allow you to turn difficult moments into opportunities for learning and connection, now and for many years ahead.

Playing with your baby

Babies learn about the world by exploring on their own and by playing with others. You are your baby's first playmate.

In the first few weeks your baby is not yet ready to play in the traditional sense, but he will intently study your face, listen to your voice, and feel your touch and your warmth. This is the time for you both to adjust and to begin getting to know each other.

Sometime in the second month you will see your baby's first true social smile. Try **taking turns smiling**. Such turn-taking is one of the earliest examples of social play that forms the foundation for interaction and language.[285] It tells your baby "I see you. You can get my attention not only by crying, but also by smiling, and I will smile back."

At first your baby will be able to play with you only for short periods of time before needing a break. When she's had enough stimulation she will stop meeting your gaze, turn away, or squirm. As you watch your baby and get to know her temperament and needs, you will learn how much playful interaction she enjoys and begin to recognize when she's ready for a break.

Soon after the first social smiles your baby will begin to experiment with sounds: cooing and babbling. Listen to your baby's vocalizations and take turns "talking." Tell your baby what you are doing and seeing as you go through the day. Remember that babies begin understanding words by about five months old—much before they utter their own first words—and that they learn language best from humans in the real world, not from screens. One of the best predictors of language development is how adults **respond to baby-initiated "conversations" and curiosity**: baby's gaze, object exploration, and, later on, gestures such as pointing and reaching.[336] As you respond to what your baby is paying attention to, your words connect to real-world objects and activities and are easier for your baby to learn. Babies whose parents support their interests and attention tend to grow into toddlers who cooperate more during daily routines, use words more, play independently for longer periods of time, and use toys in more complex ways.[256]

A wide variety of programs, books, and classes on **baby sign language** have been developed in the last two decades. There's no solid scientific evidence that learning signs benefits language development in typically developing children with normal hearing; at the same time, published studies don't report any adverse effects of sign language.[337] Teaching your baby sign language is not necessary, but if you want to do it, sign language can become an additional way for your baby to play an active role in communication.

Sing to your baby and **play music** to her. Even very young babies are sensitive to the pitch and rhythmic patterning of music and can remember tunes they hear regularly.[338] Rhythmic, faster tempo play songs are likely to capture your baby's attention during playtime. (Constant background music, however, can be overstimulating.) Singing or playing soothing lullabies may calm your baby and smooth out transitions. Singing lullabies is an ancient art found in most cultures. You may find yourself instinctually singing to your baby. If singing doesn't come naturally to you, do give it a try—and don't worry about whether you're a "good" singer, you're guaranteed to be your baby's favourite! You'll likely find singing calming for your baby and for yourself.

You have probably heard that it's important to **read** to your child, and that starting early promotes learning and future academic success. Indeed, it is never too early to share a book with your baby, although not necessarily with academic success in mind. It will take your baby a few months to begin comprehending some of the words, and quite a few more months to begin understanding the sequences of events and following storylines. But even very young babies enjoy the closeness with a family member, repetition, and experience with sounds that comes from reading and looking at a book[339]—all of which benefits cognitive and social-emotional development. Reading during the first year is not yet about content, so there's no need to read from cover-to-cover or in the correct order. Books with only a few words or with no words at all—for example, touch-and-feel board books and books with colourful illustrations of everyday objects—are great to explore with your baby. You can simply point at pictures and talk about the objects and the colours. That being said, your baby will be happy to look at the same books for several years, so you may want to choose, from the start, some stories you and your baby will enjoy reading together later on. Short, simple, positive stories are wonderful options. My babies especially enjoyed books that depicted babies, animals, and everyday objects and events they could recognize.

Book Ideas for
Babyhood and Beyond

All the World by Liz Garton Scanlon and Marla Frazee
Counting Kisses by Karen Katz
Goodnight Moon by Margaret Wise Brown
Guess How Much I Love You by Sam McBratney
Everywhere Babies by Susan Meyers
The Lion and the Bird by Marianne Dubuc
No Matter What by Debi Gliori
Peepo! by Janet and Allan Ahlberg

Offer your baby regular opportunities for **tummy time**. Spending time on her tummy will help her develop head control and core strength.[279] Many babies resist tummy time when placed alone on the floor but enjoy it as part of playing with a parent. Try positioning yourself in front of your baby face-to-face or lying on your back and placing her on your chest.

There are many **games** you can play with your older baby: peekaboo, pat-a-cake, rolling a ball, blowing bubbles, puppet shows, and building block towers, to name a few. When you offer your baby toys and play objects like blocks, balls, or stacking cups, let him initiate and choose the direction of play. Follow his lead and his interests. Babies are more likely to learn how an object works when they show interest in it first, before an adult responds and demonstrates its function.[249] You could also let your baby discover how the toy works on his own—and he might surprise you by figuring out a completely different way of playing with it! Your baby might also throw the toy you have offered him or simply take everything out of a toy basket. This is not necessarily a sign of disinterest; he might be learning about gravity and spatial concepts like "inside" and "outside."

If you love active play—for example, flying your baby like an airplane or bouncing him on your knee—be mindful of not having him become a prop in your game; watch his responses and let him be an active participant. Remember the study that showed that when parents routinely allow babies to lead in play, babies show neural activity indicative of stronger early brain development?[270] Match the intensity and timing of playful interactions to your baby's cues and stop when your baby looks tired, overstimulated, or no longer interested. Your sensitivity will give your baby opportunities to practise physiological balance, which will make it easier for him to stay calm and return to a calm state as he grows.[41]

Many adults are naturally drawn to tickling babies because it makes babies laugh. However, laughter doesn't always equal enjoyment and delight—laughing in response to tickling is our bodies' involuntary response, much like sneezing. Your baby might laugh but, unlike an older child, will not be able to tell you when she wants you to stop. There are gentler ways of bonding with your baby through touch. For example, many babies enjoy gentle infant **massage**, which has been shown to improve sleep and help relaxation and bonding.[340] There are many online resources and in-person classes available to help you learn safe infant massage techniques. The best time to offer your baby a massage is when she is calm and alert. Tell your baby what you're going to do and move slowly. Babies find it stressful to be touched without interaction; a study mentioned in Chapter 1 showed that when babies were massaged by a caregiver who made eye contact and spoke soothingly, the babies' stress hormone levels dropped, but when they were massaged in silence and without eye contact, their stress hormone levels increased.[16] Watch your baby to see whether she finds massage relaxing or stimulating and follow her lead. And last but not least, you can never go overboard with simply holding and cuddling your baby.

Connected caregiving and play ensure your baby experiences sensitivity, mind-mindedness, and positive interactions with supportive adults. As we learned in Part I of this chapter, these are important for social-emotional and cognitive development. Let's now consider the last building block of the care and play environment: free movement and exploration.

Free movement and exploration

The way your baby moves naturally is the best and safest way for him to move. When a baby has plenty of opportunities for free movement, it's easier for him to map out his own body, to gradually gain strength and awareness to prepare for sitting, crawling, and walking, and to achieve these physical milestones when he's ready.

Supporting natural motor development

It's exciting (and sometimes bittersweet!) to see your baby achieve physical milestones. Celebrate them, but try to not rush the next one. If you have concerns about your baby's motor development, be sure to discuss your concerns with your baby's health care practitioner. Otherwise, try not to worry about what your baby is not yet doing. Instead, notice what your baby can do, what she's mastering, and *how* she's moving. For example, a nine-month-old who is not crawling yet, but can go from sitting to hands-and-knees and rocking back and forth is doing exactly what she needs to do. She is getting ready for crawling by strengthening her core, leg, and arm muscles, learning to shift her weight and coordinate her limbs, and practising balancing on her hands and knees.

There are several ways you can support your baby's natural motor development:

✓ Choose clothes that allow free movement. A baby who is learning to roll or crawl and gets caught in her dress or too-long overalls can get confused and discouraged.

✓ Don't immediately rescue your baby when he's struggling to master a new skill (such as rolling) and appears frustrated. As long as he's safe, just move close and watch him carefully. He might succeed at what he's trying to do; if he doesn't succeed this time, he'll have exercised his muscles and coordination. Help him immediately if he gets into an unsafe position or location.

✓ Avoid putting your baby into positions she's not developmentally ready for. For example, don't prop her up before she's ready to sit; once she develops sufficient core strength, upper body strength, and balance, she'll get herself into a sitting position on her own.

✓ Remember that crawling is beneficial for gross and fine motor skills and for brain development. Encourage crawling by supporting your baby's pre-crawling skills: offer her regular tummy time and opportunities to play on her back and sides, don't prop her up, and allow her to move freely as much as possible so she gets comfortable moving into and out of various positions on her own. At the same time, remember that some babies naturally skip the crawling stage, and it's perfectly normal.

✓ Once your baby becomes mobile, you can offer him play equipment or household objects for safe climbing, holding on to, and crawling through: for example, sturdy couch cushions, a folding gym mat, a crawl-through tunnel, or a climbing structure designed for babies such as the Pikler triangle.

Allowing free movement is easier when you have a designated safe play area in your home. You may want to create a safe play area before your baby begins to roll or crawl. This way you'll get into the habit of observing your baby and letting her explore uninterrupted, and she'll grow to recognize this familiar, comfortable space before she's mobile.

Practical Tips for Introducing Your Baby to a Safe Play Area

It is best to introduce your baby to the safe play area when she's well-rested and not hungry. Regardless of how old your baby is, you can begin by telling her about the new space you created and showing her around; then, place her down on a flat surface, in a position that allows her to move freely. If your baby is old enough to be interested in play objects, put a few within her reach. Sit quietly beside her and watch what she chooses to do. After a while, you can begin leaving the play area. Always remain nearby so you can respond whenever your baby needs you.

Having a safe play area will allow you to rely less on baby equipment like swings or bouncy chairs. There's nothing inherently wrong with such equipment (with a couple of exceptions mentioned in Part I: baby walkers and loudly vibrating seats). Negative effects of "container" equipment—swings, bouncy chairs, exersaucers, moulded seats, baby jumpers—can occur when they're used too much. The concern is about what baby is *not* doing while spending time in a "container": she's not kicking, wiggling, turning, rolling over, balancing, sitting up, crawling, or walking. It's also hard for her to fully turn toward something interesting she hears or sees—remember, she needs to do so with her head and torso fully aligned with the direction of her gaze. Baby equipment constrains movement and sensory integration, and time spent in such equipment can add up quickly.

Eight-month-old Kai woke up, had breakfast in his high chair, and played in an exersaucer activity centre. After his morning nap he went shopping with Mom; he stayed in his car seat at the grocery store. Back home, he had lunch and an afternoon nap, and went for a stroller walk with Mom and Dad in the early evening. After dinner, Dad placed him tummy-down on a blanket on the floor and offered him some toys, but Kai quickly got frustrated as the toys kept rolling away and he couldn't reach them; Mom moved him to a bouncy seat from where he watched Mom and Dad wash dishes. Kai then had a bath playing in the water in his bath seat, and went to bed.

Kai had a nice, typical day. However, notice how much time he spent in "containers" and how little free movement he had. His opportunities to wiggle and stretch were largely limited to the times he was picked up for feeding, dressing, and diaper changes. He is likely most comfortable in a seated position because that's how he spends most of his time. He got discouraged when placed on the floor because playing there required strength and the ability to shift between positions, something he hasn't had enough opportunities to practise. Understandably, he didn't move much and protested until he was placed in a familiar seated position.

For most modern families, it's not possible to completely avoid "containers": your baby must always be buckled safely in a car seat when travelling in a vehicle; a walk in a stroller or a baby carrier can be a wonderful part of your family's daily routine; and there's nothing wrong with placing your baby in a baby seat or swing from time to time. However, try to be moderate and intentional in how much you use such equipment. Consider giving your baby plenty of opportunities for free movement, especially on days when she has to spend a considerable amount of time in the car or stroller.

Supporting free exploration

Creating a safe play area, offering your baby a selection of open-ended toys and play objects, and making time for unhurried, undirected play is all you need to do to encourage your baby to explore and experiment. He will do the rest.

Watch your baby play without setting any direction for him. When he is content and engaged in exploring a toy or mastering a new skill, sit beside him and notice what he's doing. Try to simply observe without having any particular goal in mind. What is he interested in? What might he be learning today? What is hard for him? What does he do (and how might he be feeling) when he encounters a challenge? You might choose to sit quietly or to verbally reflect back what you see ("You did it. That looked difficult"). It can be hard to stop and simply observe, as it might feel like you're doing nothing. But you're actually doing something very important: you're giving your baby your time and undivided attention. Watching your baby play is a wonderful way to practice mind-mindedness, one of the key parenting skills that promote attachment.

In addition to experimenting with toys and play objects, your baby will be exploring her own abilities: the different ways she can move and the various sounds and gestures she can make.

"Is everything all right?" my mom asked on the phone. "It sounds like a pre-historic bird..."

*Our five-month-old had found her strong voice. She prac-
tised "the screech" every waking hour for three weeks. It was
hard on my ears, but I could sense her delight so clearly that I
chose to not distract or redirect her. It became one of the many
skills she discovered by herself and practised joyfully and confidently. (I won't lie, though: I was relieved when she moved on
to practising how to push herself up to a sitting position!)*

Give your baby regular opportunities to experiment and
explore uninterrupted. This will help your baby's motor skills
and cognitive development, including her ability to pay focused
attention. Last but not least, it will support her growing sense of
mastery and competence.

This concludes the last building block of the care and play
environment you can create in your home. However, your growing baby will also be spending time out in the world: meeting
and visiting people, joining you during outings, and, perhaps,
attending playgroups or daycare. During the early months and
years we, parents and caregivers, still have the power to influence
baby's environment outside of our home by making intentional
choices.

At home in the world

New people and experiences

Babies meet lots of new people and have many new experiences
during their first year. How they react partially depends on their
temperaments. Outgoing babies tend to approach anything unfamiliar with curiosity, while more cautious, slower-to-warm-up
babies tend to withdraw or hesitate at first. This characteristic
is something your baby was born with. But it's not necessarily
an indication of how he will approach new people and events

when he grows up, because his life experiences will join his temperament in shaping his unique personality. If your baby's temperament is quite different from your own, try to recognize and accept the differences. Neither is better or worse; each temperament comes with its own strengths and challenges.

Regardless of your baby's temperament, around the age of seven to nine months he is likely to begin showing *stranger anxiety* (fear of strangers and unfamiliar events) and *separation anxiety* (reluctance to separate from you). As you may recall, by this age babies develop:[25]

- ✓ Focused attachment ("I know who brings me love, safety, and nourishment")
- ✓ Understanding of object permanence ("That person with big glasses is still in the kitchen although I cannot see her")
- ✓ Advanced ability to detect patterns and anticipate events ("Mommy has her coat on so she must be leaving")

These cognitive leaps expand your baby's world, but also make it appear more uncertain, so he might cling to his safe base more tightly. In addition, babies at this age are gaining, or are about to gain, mobility. Stranger and separation anxiety might serve as a safety net that keeps them closer to parents and caregivers.

Here is how you can help your baby navigate the unfamiliar:

- Tell your baby ahead of time about the new person he will soon be meeting ("My friend Katie is coming to see us after lunch"). Remember, babies begin to understand words early.
- Avoid labels when you talk to your baby or introduce him to someone (instead of saying "Oh, he's just shy," try saying "Aidan is learning to meet new people" or "Aidan needs extra time today").

- Respect your baby's cautiousness or fear, but don't reinforce it (instead of "this vacuum *is* scary!" try "I see you feel scared").
- Make time for your baby to warm up to a new person or situation; don't pass him to anyone to hold or hug before he is ready.
- When you're about to leave your baby with a family member or a caregiver, don't slip away quietly: tell your baby that you're leaving, and that you'll be back soon.

Stranger and separation anxiety usually lasts a few months, sometimes longer. These behaviours are developmentally appropriate and are a testament to your baby's strong bond with you. Overcoming them requires cognitive and emotional development and repeated experiences. Watching you interact with people will help your baby become more comfortable doing it herself. And having small, natural separations during the day ("I'm going to the kitchen; I'll see you in a minute") will gradually teach her that you always come back.

Baby groups and classes

Despite what advertisers might tell you, your baby does not *need* extracurricular activities: he will have plenty of natural learning opportunities spending time with you at home and accompanying you on walks, errands, and visits with people in your life. When you hear of a baby group or a class that piques your interest, ask yourself these questions:

- Does this opportunity fit well into my baby's daily rhythm (won't interfere with sleep, does not require hours spent in the car)?

- Is this something I would personally like to do? Is it likely to help me on my parenting journey by giving *me* opportunities to learn, socialize, connect, or expand my circle?

If you answered "yes" to both questions, the class is worth considering. Watch your baby's signals to see when (and if) he's ready to be brought into a structured activity. Sometimes your baby might benefit more from observing others do it or even watching something else happening in the room. As Magda Gerber puts it in *Your Self-Confident Baby*, "for babies, being who they are is the curriculum."[341]

Daycare

If you plan to return to work, you will have important decisions to make as you select and arrange for care for your baby. It's natural to have doubts and worries about this process; they show the depth of your love for your baby and the strength of your sense of responsibility. However, don't let these doubts keep you from starting your search early. Where I live, the demand for daycare is so high that parents have to put their names on waitlists before their babies are born, and sometimes even before conception. Although your situation may be different, consider starting your search early so you have choices and can select one that fits best. No daycare arrangement will be absolutely perfect, but with time and effort you will find the best possible solution, one you and your baby are both comfortable with.

You'll have many factors to consider: for example, whether to choose a large daycare centre, a family daycare, or a nanny; location, hours, and cost; accreditation type; child care philosophy; staff training; the immunization policy; and parent involvement. Some of these factors may be more important to you than others depending on your circumstances. But science tells us that **the**

most important factor for your baby (after physical safety) **is a consistent, attentive, and loving caregiver.** Every baby needs loving responsiveness from a small core of adults in her life, especially in situations that are uncertain or stressful. We saw in Part I that babies have higher stress levels at daycare compared to home even months after they settle in. (That being said, remember they are experiencing stress, but may or may not be affected by it.) It'll be essential for your baby to form an attachment relationship with her caregiver: a close, loving bond.

When you interview a home-based daycare provider or nanny, look for signs that they understand and value attachment and will make a commitment to connect with your baby, in addition to providing safety and meeting the baby's needs for sleep and nutrition. Does the caregiver see babies as unique individuals to get to know and develop a bond with?

In choosing a daycare centre, ask whether the centre practices **primary caregiving** where one caregiver consistently takes care of a small group of babies (as opposed to all staff watching all babies). Ask questions. Does the centre have high staff turnover? Does it implement rotating shifts where multiple caregivers take care of babies throughout the course of each day or week? Does the centre rely heavily on student workers? If babies move to a different room within the centre as they grow, does their primary caregiver move with them (an approach called looping)? Having continuity of care—a special, key person at daycare who knows your baby well—will help your baby join in the daycare routines, feel more comfortable, and have an easier time with transitions like moving rooms and meeting new children.

Consider interviewing several caregivers and visiting several daycare centres in person. Ask not only for a visit with the centre's director, but also for an opportunity to quietly observe various activities around the centre. This will help you get a feel for how the different written philosophies and policies translate into everyday practices. Something that looks great on paper may not be so in real life, and the other way around.

 Choosing a Daycare
Centre: What to Look For

Does the centre:

- ✓ ensure a low children-to-teacher ratio?
- ✓ value and practise primary caregiving where one care-giver consistently takes care of a small group of babies?
- ✓ promote openness and communication with parents?
- ✓ have a vision that matches the values of your family?

Do the caregivers:

- ✓ connect with individual children?
- ✓ recognize the need for babies to have individual daily rhythms, as opposed to one schedule for all?
- ✓ appear well-supported in their jobs?

Does the daycare environment have:

- ✓ safe, clean, separate areas for sleep, eating, diapering, and play?
- ✓ a calm atmosphere (not too loud or bright)?
- ✓ safe spaces to move, indoors and outdoors?
- ✓ simple, interesting materials to explore?

Visiting in person will allow you to see the interactions between caregivers and babies. Note whether the caregivers speak directly to the babies or only to each other. Do they give each baby their full attention during feeding and diaper changes or do they rush through to get the job done? Daycares often have daily schedules posted for parents to see. Ask if they offer flexibility in accommodating babies' individual daily rhythms: for example, are babies provided with opportunities to rest when they're tired or do they have to wait until a set nap time? Honouring individual babies' sleep rhythms requires a separate, well-ventilated, dark area for sleep and rest; some daycares don't have such an area and just convert the playroom to nap room once a day on a schedule, which is not ideal for meeting the sleep needs of young children.

Science tells us that for babies, the overall environment is more important than specific learning activities. Does the daycare setup feel clean, calm, and nurturing? Look for uncluttered spaces, fresh air, indirect lighting, and noise control. Do the babies have spaces to move, indoors and outdoors? It's not necessary to have educational programming or any sort of curriculum. Are the babies you observe pushed to learn or are they free to play and explore?

Some daycares follow specific educational philosophies, like Montessori, Waldorf, or Reggio Emilia, or adopt elements from several of them. These centres may be a wonderful fit for your baby and family, but remember that daycares, even if they derive from the same philosophy, can be quite different from one another. What's most important are caring relationships and a safe, calm environment.

Once you've chosen a daycare, plan to settle your baby in gradually; the transition might take time. Prepare a one-page note describing your baby's routines at home and share it with the caregiver before your baby's first day. Send in a familiar blanket or a sleep-safe cuddle toy if your baby has one. Share your beliefs and any concerns you have; don't assume that the caregivers have seen it all and know everything. Supportive care for your baby will require both their knowledge (of babies in general) and your knowledge (of your unique baby). Let the daycare know you want to help foster the bond between your baby and her primary caregiver, and ask for their recommendations and support.

When your baby begins attending daycare, help her stay as well-rested at home as possible. It might be tempting to keep her up late so you have more time together in the evenings. But remember that babies and toddlers who sleep soundly at home have lower cortisol at daycare compared to those who don't sleep well.[315] Sleeping well at home will help your baby feel more comfortable at daycare.

Care and play stories

A safe space

The problem was the Lego®. Well, not the Lego itself, but all the tiny pieces that five-year-old Sawyer loved playing with on the family room floor where eight-month-old Ben would scoop them up and try to put them in his mouth. Ben also instantly found every little crumb in the kitchen. To address the issue, the boys' dad began by adding a low bookshelf to Sawyer's room (a "special home for Lego"). A week later he added a large play yard made with interlocked gates to the family room: a safe play area for Ben. The rest of the family room was "family space" where they could spend time together while watching Ben closely. Ben's play area initially included a set of stacking cups, a ball, a couple of cloth books, and a folded gym mat (new to Ben). He loved climbing on and off the gym mat, which helped with the transition. As Ben grew, his play area grew with him: his parents added board books, trucks, dolls, and a simple play kitchen. Ben and Sawyer's grandparents enjoyed giving gifts to the kids so there were several sets of toys to rotate. Ben had his play space until he turned three years old.

My cautious baby

Many people remarked that Leah was a very alert baby. She was observant and, because of that, easily overstimulated. By the time she was six months old, I'd figured out that she needed more than the average amount of sleep to be well-rested. I made several adjustments to our daily rhythm at home and chose to stop attending a mid-morning mom-and-baby group. This group gave me an opportunity to meet other parents, but Leah was tired from missing her morning nap and not keen to participate in group activities most of the time. (I later found another parenting circle through our local library that aligned with Leah's naps well—and we both enjoyed it.)

When Leah was around eight months old, she became very cautious when she met new people or had new experiences. One evening a friend visited us for dinner; he had a long beard, something Leah had never seen before. Leah appeared scared at first and spent most of the evening watching from the safety of our arms. We chose to not push her to interact with our guest or play independently, but she eventually did both.

We don't have family living nearby, but we wanted Leah to be familiar with close family members when we visited. Part of her bedtime routine included looking at a picture gallery in our hallway on the way to her bedroom, talking about the people we love, and saying goodnight to them.

We chose to have no television or other screen time apart from an occasional video call for Leah (and later, Tessa) for the first four years. This may seem unrealistic, but it wasn't difficult for us: even before kids came along we didn't have cable television, and we deliberately limited internet access to a desktop computer in our home office since we both use screens throughout our work days.

As I write this, we are in the midst of the COVID-19 pandemic. Schools are closed, and Leah, who is now eight, is confidently using a desktop and a tablet for remote learning. She has a close-knit group of friends, and she eagerly embraces the majority of new experiences and opportunities. She still needs more than an average amount of sleep. I sometimes catch myself alerting the kids when I am about to use a noisy coffee grinder, which is now all but a reminder of Leah's babyhood and toddler years.

Questions you may have

Q The idea of using gates to block off a play space feels restrictive and prison-like to me. Won't my baby feel trapped?

A I like to think of the gates forming a safe play area in the same way I think about the harnesses in babies' car seats, strollers, or high chairs: they allow babies to have new experiences (a car ride, a walk, practice in self-feeding) by keeping them safe and secure. A safe play area where your baby is free to explore can, in fact, be less restrictive than a typical room where many objects are not okay to touch, mouth, or climb on.

Q Our daycare recommended brief timeouts for our eleven-month-old so she can learn not to pull on adults' glasses and hair. Is this a good idea?

A Although a timeout is arguably a better option than old-school punishment, timeouts don't teach babies anything useful. Your baby is unlikely to understand that being taken to another room and left alone is linked to her trying to pull someone's glasses off. In addition, the timeout may not feel "brief" to her because she doesn't yet have a concept of time. A timeout in a crib or a play area—somewhat natural choices due to safety—is confusing for babies, as it contradicts the familiar patterns ("Am I supposed to sleep?") and, over time, may lead them to protest spending time in these spaces. A better approach would be to set a boundary ("Grandma needs her glasses. Please don't pull on them."). If your baby continues to try, gently but firmly take her in your arms and hold her if she's upset. Later, show your baby how to touch your hair or a toy gently without pulling. This approach links the consequences with the behaviour naturally and fosters connection rather than isolation.

There is, however, one important exception where a time-out is necessary: when you are overwhelmed to a point where you might not act rationally and *you* need a timeout. In this case it is best to place your baby in the crib or a safe area, take a deep breath, call someone, and arrange for help.

Watch and Wonder

There will be many times when you won't know why your baby is crying. Check for immediate needs and discomforts first; if she's still crying, hold her and allow her to continue crying as you keep listening and observing.

Babies can understand words they hear often. If your baby is five months or older, what words might he already know?

One day your baby will initiate his own game with you. Try to capture it on video next time it happens or write about it in your baby's journal if you have one.

Developmental milestones are guides and ranges, not rules. If your baby's health care practitioner is not concerned, don't worry or focus on upcoming milestones: try to notice and soak up what your baby *is* doing. Meet your baby where she is in her development. What can you do to "scaffold" her natural learning process? How can you give her just the right amount of support to encourage mastery?

The final chapter of this book is not about your baby; rather, it is about someone incredibly important to your baby: you.

CHAPTER 5
YOUR ROLE

"We don't get to practice for parenthood"
— Laura Davis and Janis Keyser,
Becoming the Parent You Want to Be

D id you know that the use of "parent" as a verb is a relatively new phenomenon? It was only in the 1970s that this word began shifting from a noun (something you *are*) to a verb (something you *do*).[342] Of course, adults have been raising children for millennia, but over the last few decades being a parent has come to mean not only providing and caring for children, but also actively shaping them so they turn out "right."[3] Modern science has shown us that not everything is determined by our babies' genetic makeup; we now know that care and nurturing—things we have control over—make a significant difference.

This knowledge is empowering, but it also comes with a heavy sense of responsibility. We live in a time of conscious, and some would say hyperconscious, parenting. We want to parent well; we have high expectations for ourselves and society expects a lot of us, too. At the same time, most of us no longer have a "village": an extended family or community that provides us with an intuitive base that comes from seeing how babies are raised and links new parents into a circle of support. Our society isn't always set up to support parents. Many of us have to return to work in the early months or even weeks of our baby's life, we work long hours, and we have difficulty finding quality daycare. We often find ourselves amidst fear-mongering and finger-pointing, but without reliable information and support. We may be fortunate to have many options, but it's often hard to choose, and nothing seems enough. We begin focusing on problems instead of seeing the big picture and all the things that are going well.

In this final chapter, I've gathered scientific findings that challenge several common beliefs about parenthood and parenting knowledge, beliefs that shape what we expect of ourselves as parents and what we expect of others who walk this path beside us. I hope this information helps you feel more confident and supported in your role as a parent or caregiver.

PART I
PARENTING KNOWLEDGE: THE SCIENCE

Each person and every family experience the transition into parenthood in their own unique way, which is difficult to put into words. For me, the transition was rewarding, challenging, and life-altering. Similarly, what parenting is made of—love, responsibility, devotion, sacrifice, joy—is difficult to describe and even more difficult to study. But science does provide answers to several questions that most new parents wonder about. How will I know what to do once my baby is here? Do mothers naturally know how to raise babies? Should I trust expert advice or my gut feelings? And, ultimately: what are our most important roles as parents?

Maternal instinct

You have likely heard of the concept of "maternal instinct": an idea that women naturally know how to take care of babies and children. Maternal instinct is believed to switch on as soon as a woman becomes a mother, making her innately better at parenting than the father and other caregivers. Are women indeed predisposed to knowing how to care for babies—and do men lack that predisposition? Science says no, this is not the case. Maternal instinct as a magical set of skills and knowledge available to mothers simply does not exist.

What does exist is a *caregiving drive* (or "parental care motivational system," as scientists call it). Neuroscience has shown that seeing babies' faces and hearing babies cry activates two powerful desires in human adults:

1. A desire to nurture, which makes us tender, empathetic, selfless, and caring
2. A desire to protect, which makes us alert, careful, and risk averse

Together, these form the caregiving drive. Caregiving drive is part of human nature and is universal: it is present regardless of a parent's gender, sexual orientation, or age. It is activated in mothers and fathers[343-348] across cultures.[35] Moreover, adults who are not parents themselves show similar brain activation patterns in response to babies. These brain patterns emerge in just a hundred milliseconds, which tells us they are subconscious: they don't require rational thinking, they just happen.[347]

This powerful, universal, biology-based, subconscious caregiving drive makes all of us—mothers, fathers, and other committed caregivers—*want* to care for our babies the best we can. However, what it doesn't do is tell us *how*; we have to figure that out ourselves, using evidence-based knowledge and our intuition.

Evidence-based knowledge

Evidence-based parenting knowledge is the facts, information, and skills we get by learning, thinking, and understanding. It's no surprise that parenting knowledge increases parents' competence and is associated with better child development and health outcomes.[349] Surveys suggest that first-time parents want to learn more about parenting and child development, but they have difficulty obtaining clear and trustworthy advice; the amount of information is overwhelming and its quality is inconsistent.[350]

Seeking advice from trusted health care professionals and solid scientific studies—as we've done throughout this book—allows us to "find the signal through the noise" in the form of reliable, evidence-based knowledge.

Intuition

If maternal instinct is largely a myth, why do so many mothers and fathers show a strong sense of *just knowing* when something is wrong (or right) with their children? This "sixth sense" or "gut feeling"—our *intuition*—indeed exists. But it doesn't switch on as soon as we become parents either.

The word "intuition" comes from the Latin verb *intuēri*, which means *to look upon* or *to see from within*. Historically, psychologists have been reluctant to acknowledge intuition as a real phenomenon, but it has now been documented by research. Intuition gives us the ability to know something directly without analytic reasoning, without weighing the facts. In contrast with conscious and deliberate evidence-based knowledge, intuition is subconscious and automatic. Essentially, intuition is a way of knowing without being able to explain how we know.

Intuition is a true form of knowledge, because it comes from the way our brains store, process, and retrieve memories.[351, 352] In essence, we subconsciously call on information from past experiences stored in our memory and combine it to draw new conclusions.[353] Highly intuitive people extract the maximum amount of significance from the available information, because they see meaning in details others may overlook.

So intuition is the synthesis of the experiences we carry within us, but where do these experiences come from? In the context of raising babies, they could be the product of:

- Careful observation

- Our culture
- Biases and fads

These three sources are not equally reliable. Depending on the source, intuition can be accurate, but it also can be very wrong.[354]

Careful observation

Our first source of intuitive knowledge is our unique babies. We develop intuition as we spend time with them and get to know them better than anyone else. To date, very little research has specifically focused on intuition in the context of raising children. Intuitive parenting is described in the scientific literature as "the non-conscious parental behaviours that offer developmental support and are highly adapted to serve the best interests of the infant." Examples include parents speaking directly to their babies, adjusting their distances based on how far babies can see, and fine-tuning their caregiving according to babies' need for stimulation.[355] Other studies that weren't specifically focused on parenting intuition documented positive effects of tuning in and observing babies. Throughout this book you saw many examples of how careful observation can help parents get to know their babies and understand their needs—and how doing so allows babies' natural development to unfold. Small observations accumulate to form our special intuitive knowledge of our babies.

The Benefits of Careful Observation: Examples

✓ Learning babies' sleep cues (such as slight quieting, staring off, calmness, a lull in energy) helps prevent overtiredness and supports natural sleep development, so babies can begin sleeping as soundly as they can as early as they are ready (Chapter 2).

✓ Learning babies' hunger cues helps us see whether they are hungry or have another need such as the need to be comforted. Responding to babies sensitively—feeding them when they're hungry, comforting them when they're upset—helps preserve their innate ability to eat to appetite and to continue tuning into their sensations as they grow (Chapter 3).

✓ Watching for signs of readiness for solid foods allows us to offer solids within the best developmental window, which helps babies master different tastes and textures more easily and allows them to enjoy the early meals more (Chapter 3).

✓ Observing babies as they play supports their developing attention and encourages independent exploration, cooperation during caregiving routines, communication, and problem solving (Chapter 4).

Culture

The second source intuition can draw upon is our cultural values and beliefs. Culture, along with genes, is the main kind of information passed down from one generation to the next.[356] Culture differs across societies in different parts of the world and can also differ among groups within one society. In relation to parenting, scientists commonly classify cultures into two categories:

1. Cultures that predominantly value independence: autonomy, self-sufficiency, and freedom to act on personal choices

2. Cultures that predominantly value connected interdependence: being part of a larger system of relationships, loyalty, respect for hierarchy, and collective achievements

These values are not necessarily mutually exclusive or opposite: for all of us, self-sufficiency, freedom, duty, and loyalty are important in certain situations at certain times in our lives. But in general, cultures do appear to have dominant values and goals,[357] and parents consciously and subconsciously use these culturally constructed values in raising their children. For example, American society is commonly characterized as one that values independence, whereas Japanese society values connected interdependence. Consequently, American and Japanese parents tend to work toward somewhat different goals:[357, 358] American mothers try to promote autonomy, assertiveness, and verbal competence in their children, whereas Japanese mothers try to promote emotional maturity, self-control, empathy, compliance, and understanding of social cues and norms. And these values influence day-by-day caregiving.

Differences in parenting approaches between cultures[357, 358]

Cultures that value independence	Cultures that value interdependence
Respond to crying babies promptly	Respond to babies proactively by anticipating their needs (before they cry)
Bond and communicate through face-to-face interaction using words and gestures	Bond and communicate through physical closeness, touch, and facial expressions
Respond to challenging behaviour by reasoning and encouraging independent thinking	Respond to challenging behaviour using physical positioning and direct requests

Despite these differences, the mutual connection between parents and their babies is similar across cultures. Even if caregiving looks different in families with different backgrounds, it can still be sensitive and well-suited to meeting babies' needs.[357]

Cultures also differ in routines and rituals, sleep arrangements, traditional foods, and many other aspects of daily life. In this book I focused on the fundamental abilities and needs of all human babies and the universal elements of the Optimal Nurturing Environment (the ONE) that helps babies reach their full potential. The universal nature of these elements means that families can create them in a number of different ways that reflect, incorporate, and honour their cultural backgrounds.

Incorporating Culture Into Babies' Environments: Examples

✓ All babies benefit from sound sleep. Typical bedtimes for babies and toddlers vary greatly across cultures—from 7:30 p.m. to 10:20 p.m.—but all young children wake up early, generally between 6 and 8 a.m. (page 34). To make sure their babies get enough sleep, families can choose an earlier bedtime than customary in their community or offer their babies more opportunities for daytime naps (being mindful, however, that babies don't fully catch up on sleep by napping more[97, 120]).

✓ All babies have tiny tummies and grow and develop incredibly fast, thus requiring highly nutrient-dense foods (pages 117–120). One of the critically important nutrients is iron, which can be incorporated into babies' diets in a variety of ways. For example, some families may primarily rely on red meat, poultry, and eggs, while others on fish, beans, lentils, spinach, and fortified cereals.

✓ All babies benefit from exploration and play. Traditional toys and play objects vary across cultures, but all are great options as long as they're safe and, ideally, open-ended (i.e., can be used in a variety of ways).

Parenting within culture can help create environments that are positive, consistent, predictable, and similar to what children are likely to encounter outside their family as they grow. However, acting upon intuitions that stem from cultural beliefs without supplementing them with conscious reasoning—without checking them against evidence-based knowledge—can lead us astray. For example, a cultural belief that babies are born "blank slates" (which science has clearly shown to be untrue) could lead to parents not noticing their baby's unique abilities and temperament. This could expose her to overstimulation and impact early attachment.

Biases and fads

Finally, what we consider intuition can also be what Po Bronson and Ashley Merryman in *NurtureShock* call "a hodgepodge of wishful thinking, moralistic biases, contagious fads, personal history, and old (disproven) psychology."[359] Our memories are cluttered with mixed messages from the media, fads, implicit biases, and peer pressure, and we might subconsciously use these in what we think is intuitive decision-making. Such intuitions are really more of a conditioned response, and they're usually radically mistaken.

Combining knowledge

Recent research suggests that the human brain is able to combine intuition and external evidence-based knowledge even when we're not aware of the source of the intuition.[360] So it's beneficial to listen to our intuition *and* deliberately and carefully consider evidence-based knowledge before making decisions. That process makes us more likely to filter out irrelevant cultural messages, biases, and fads that we could have mistaken for intuition, and free us to use truly intuitive knowledge—our inner knowledge that comes from carefully observing our babies and reflects the values we believe in—wisely.

Carefully considering evidence-based information allows us to use our truly intuitive knowledge of our babies without conflating it with fads.

The work of parenthood

The 1960s, when many mothers didn't work outside the home, are sometimes thought of as family-oriented years. Today, the dual-income family is the norm, and working parents often feel guilty for not being able to spend more time at home. Yet—and you might find this surprising—studies across sixteen Western countries show that today's parents spend *more* face-to-face time with their children than those in the 1960s did.[361-363] We live with the cultural expectation of "intensive" parenting.[364] Today's parents preserve and even increase the time they devote to their children by cutting down on their own leisure activities. And the number-one such "leisure" activity is sleep.[362]

This trend—increasing the time we spend with our children—is true for both mothers and fathers. Fathers today are doing more housework and spending more time with their children than the fathers of the 1960s, '70s, and '80s. But the gender gap remains: studies consistently show that mothers are generally doing more work—and feeling more of the stress—that comes with parenthood.[362, 365]

Science points to three reasons that mothers tend to take on larger loads. The first one is public policy. Of forty-one countries surveyed by the Pew Research Center in 2018, paid leave for fathers was available in thirty-four of them, but most offered only two weeks' leave or less.[366] It can be difficult for fathers to become fully engaged when they don't spend a significant amount of time with their babies. To get truly involved and attuned, all parents—male or female, biological or adoptive—need time and practise through day-by-day caregiving. One study compared mothers' and fathers' abilities to recognize their own baby's cry among the cries of other babies. Who do you think did better? Mothers and fathers did equally well, but only if they routinely spent at least four hours a day with their baby.[345] Another study showed that in gay male couples, the primary-caregiver fathers—the partners who provided most of the baby care—had the same brain patterns as primary-caregiver mothers in heterosexual couples.[346] These studies tell us that the key to engaged parenting is not gender but the time put into—and responsibility felt for—the day-by-day caregiving.

There's another reason mothers take on a larger load. It has to do with the way housework is commonly managed within families. In general, men tend to look after non-routine tasks like yard work and repairs; such tasks are relatively flexible in terms of when they must be done. Women, however, often take care of the more routine and less flexible tasks such as cooking, cleaning, and laundry.[367] These tasks need to be done daily or multiple times a day, and often at specific times, requiring multitasking when also looking after children. Mothers, indeed, tend to multitask[368] and feel more stressed.[369]

> Multitasking is stressful because of the way the human brain handles it. In short, it doesn't! Our brains can only focus on one thing at a time. It might seem like you're accomplishing multiple things at the same time, but what you are really doing is quickly shifting your attention from one thing to the next which can be taxing—and stressful.[370]

The third reason mothers are overworked and stressed is that sometimes they themselves—usually unintentionally, sometimes unconsciously—stand in the way of partnership in parenting. They *gatekeep*, undermining and limiting their partner's opportunities for caring for the children and the home. Among dual-income, white, middle-class, metropolitan couples in the western United States, every fifth mother was classified as a gatekeeper.[371]

Mothers are likely to gatekeep when they carry all the "mental load" or "worry work" of parenthood: anticipating needs, obtaining knowledge, identifying options, making decisions, and monitoring progress, essentially acting as the project managers for the family.[372] Mothers are also more likely to gatekeep when they're anxious, when they hold excessively high expectations for the fathers' parenting, when they feel their relationship is unstable, and when fathers lack confidence.[373-375]

In summary, maternal instinct is a myth, and parenting is learned through both external knowledge (of what *all* babies need) and careful observation (of *our own* babies and families). Let's take a look at how these scientific findings can help you feel more confident and supported in your parenting, as well as support others committed to caring for your baby alongside you.

PART II
YOU

I f there were one thing I could tell my pre-motherhood self, it would be this: expect to love, and prepare to give; the rest will be different from what you envision. Nothing truly prepared me for how all-consuming, and at times overwhelming, caring for my babies would feel. In the early weeks I barely knew who I was outside of my need to be there for them.

Becoming a parent of a newborn makes you a newly born parent: an incredibly important role you have not had a chance to practise for. Your role is central. You create the environment for sleep, feeding, care, and play. You are the centre of your baby's universe, the core of the ONE. You are love.

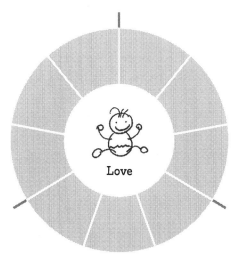

Love

The ONE approach: you are love, and your role is central.

To be a strong core, you, too, need a safe and supportive environment.

Supporting yourself and others

"A lifetime supply of insufficiency arrives with the stretch marks"
— Karen Maezen Miller, *Momma Zen*

Much happiness, love, and joy await you in parenthood. But your feelings won't all be happy ones; some days you may feel depleted, overwhelmed, tired, or lonely, or maybe even all of the above.

Practical Tip:
On Days When You're Feeling...

- **Anxious:** Your baby is lucky to have someone who cares deeply. Feeling anxious about things we can change may lead us to observing and thinking more carefully, and to learning more. Feeling fearful about things we cannot change, such as imagining all the scary things that might happen to our children, also has its purpose: it's a way to explore the strength of our connection and to accept the extent of our responsibility for another human being.[335]

- **Exhausted:** Exhaustion in parenthood comes not only from the lack of sleep, but also from the incredible amount of attention you are paying to your baby.[335] Paying careful attention takes a lot of energy. In addition, the multitasking that inevitably comes with parenthood can be exhausting.[368,369] Ask for help and look for opportunities to rest when you can; when you can't, try accepting tiredness rather than fighting it. "Be what you are... be tired."[147]

- **Overwhelmed:** Parenthood is biologically meant to overwhelm us (remember the powerful caregiving drive, and the fact that it takes our brains only a hundred milliseconds to respond to a crying baby?). As Beth Berry says in *Motherwhelmed*, overwhelm is not a sign of weakness but a sign of importance.[376] When you feel you have too much to do during the small windows when your baby is napping, try to mentally replace "I have to do so much" with "I get to do a few things I am fortunate to be doing." For example, you might think, "Today, I get to have a shower/fold laundry/make plans," or, simply, "Today, I get to hold my baby through his nap."

- **Desperate to get back to your old self:** Becoming a parent, especially for the first time, is life-changing: you not only meet your baby, but you also discover yourself as a mother or father. If you crave alone time, try to carve it out and do something that helps you feel nourished physically or emotionally: connect with a friend or family member, exercise, read, have a bath, or work on a project you've been wanting to do. When it's not possible to have alone time, try a walk with your baby in a stroller or carrier for some quiet time together. As your baby grows you'll become better rested, get more time for yourself, and have the chance to return to hobbies you enjoyed pre-baby, yet life will always be different. In some ways you'll get back to your old self, and in other ways you will go beyond that. Did you know that mothers are forever transformed by each pregnancy, and not just emotionally? During pregnancy, mother and baby exchange cells; some of the baby's cells remain in his mother's body for decades after birth, a phenomenon called microchimerism. These cells have a stem cell–like nature and may play a role in healing wounds, as they appear to flock to sites of injury.[377] So if you've carried a baby inside of you, you are now indeed a slightly different person!

- **Self-critical:** Some days we have less energy to devote to parenting than others, and all of us make mistakes. Mistakes can be good learning opportunities. Don't look at yourself from a deficit point of view. Try to see the big picture—your dedication, your hard work, your strengths—instead of zooming in on something that did not go as planned.

- **Lonely:** Being with babies and children means you are almost never alone, but sometimes lonely. The way you spend your time has changed; your circle of friends might change too. Look for like-minded parents, for friends who support and cheer you on rather than compare or judge. Help others when their babies arrive, to connect and to grow love and hope.

New parents often feel "less than." I remember a friend saying, "I'm now a mom, and I should know what I'm doing. I should be naturally good at this, but I don't think I am." In fact, what's natural—and perfectly okay—is to *not* know what to do.

The idea that one should instinctively and instantly know what to do once they become a parent is unrealistic; it can bring anxiety, stress, and a sense of failure.

Remember, there is no maternal instinct, no magically acquired knowledge. When you don't expect or count on instinct, you are free to learn and grow as a parent.

Caring for children was never meant to be done alone. For millennia across cultures, birth and postpartum has been women's work, but never the work of one woman alone. In today's families, fathers are invited to be full partners in birth and early parenting, yet many have had no role models to show them how. When a baby joins the family, sometimes the new father does not get involved enough and the mother becomes overworked and stressed. Changing social policies that contribute to this issue is going to take time, but there are certain things you can do to create a better balance within your family.

1. **Learn together**

   When only one partner carries all the mental load of parenthood—anticipating needs, obtaining knowledge, identifying options, making decisions—it can be hard for them not to impose their insights or standards on the other partner. This can lead to gatekeeping. Gatekeepers might do everything themselves or look over their partner's shoulder, giving directions and criticizing how they interact with and care for the baby. Gatekeeping can become a vicious cycle because the other partner backs off thinking they'll never get it right; they engage less with the baby and feel less and less confident. At the same time, the gatekeeper is likely to feel overworked, exhausted, alone, and as if they are responsible for any and all mistakes. To avoid gatekeeping, learn together by looking for evidence-based knowledge and by observing your baby. Share what you've learned and noticed. Take the time to discuss anything you disagree on; try to agree on big issues, especially those related to your baby's health and safety.

2. Work together—but also apart

Studies tell us that the key to engaged parenting is the time put into—and responsibility felt for—the day-to-day caregiving. Usually one partner—often, though not always, Mom—spends more time with the baby. For the primary caregiver to get a break, and for her partner to be truly involved, it helps to put some of the daily parenting tasks under the partner's full responsibility. When they consistently take care of a task—for example, dinner or bath time—without having to be asked or reminded and from start to finish, the primary caregiver can let go of the task physically and mentally. If you choose to go this route, both you and your partner need to accept that the other person might do things differently. Whoever's in charge of a task must have space to make their own decisions, not just execute the decisions made for them.

And neither partner should look over the other's shoulder or perceive their version as "less than."

3. Appreciate each other

Should you make a special effort to distribute the parenting load equally? Probably not. Yours and your partner's commitments outside your home, the needs of your baby, and your perceptions will continue to change, making it difficult, if not impossible, to be exactly the same amount of involved. What matters is how you both feel about it. When it comes to housework, it's not the unequal division of labour that causes conflict, but the lack of recognition and appreciation.[378] Perhaps the same is true for parenting. Remember to notice what your partner does and to thank them as much as possible. And when it comes to emotional work of raising children, I once heard that partners should strive not for 50:50, but for 100:100. Connect with your baby fully and love her with all your heart; notice when your partner does the same.

Your role in the ONE

In this book I focused on the needs of all human babies to describe the optimal development arena: the ONE. I walked you through its universal, set-by-biology building blocks that we now understand thanks to science.

At first glance, the building blocks of the ONE can seem complex, as they're full of options and possibilities. But these options actually make the ONE straightforward—and liberating. Each building block can be put into place in a number of ways. You will create your own unique practices that match your values and your circumstances. Once you create your practices within the ONE, you will know you are raising your baby in the biologically

optimal range that supports his unfolding abilities. You won't
need to worry whether your approaches match a particular parenting philosophy, and you won't need to measure your choices
against those of other families. You'll be free to nurture—and
apply—your intuitive knowledge.

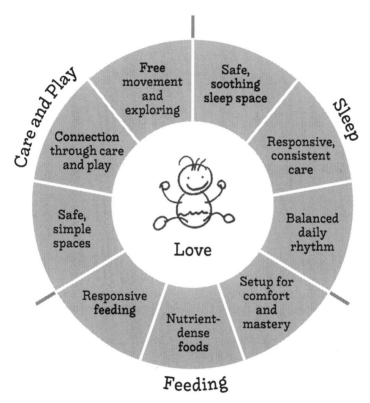

The ONE approach, complete.

The ONE also frees you from the insidious "shoulds" of parenting: putting your baby on a schedule, making your baby eat,
making sure your baby hits all the developmental milestones
right on time, keeping your baby happy, and always knowing
exactly what to do. In fact, you are not responsible for any of
these. Your role in each element of the ONE is much more realis-
tic (although not always easy):

What you are *not* responsible for	Your role
Knowing exactly what to do from the start	Growing your knowledge and nurturing your intuition
Making your baby sleep	Creating a safe space for sleep and providing responsive and consistent care
Putting your baby on a schedule	Helping your baby develop balanced internal rhythms
Making your baby eat	Providing nutritious food and a safe place and appropriate time to eat
Ensuring your baby follows the average weight curve	Feeding responsively to help your baby retain the ability to eat to appetite
Making sure your baby is always happy	Responding to your baby's needs and feelings with sensitivity and mind-mindedness
Teaching developmental milestones	Creating spaces and experiences that allow development to unfold
Ensuring your baby develops certain personality traits	Supporting your baby in being who they are and in growing into who they are meant to be
Getting the approval of others	Making decisions based on knowledge (of what all babies need and of your own unique baby)
Being a perfect parent	Loving your baby and doing your best

The last one—loving your baby and doing your best—is the most important.

EPILOGUE

Just wait

When I was a bleary-eyed and anxious new mom of a four-month-old, I asked my sister-in-law, a mom of two older children, whether life would get easier soon. "No," she replied, "it won't get easier. It'll just be different." Although I found it disheartening at the time, I now see that she gave me the most honest answer possible. We gain confidence, our babies grow and reach milestones, but new stages and new challenges will always arrive to humble us and make us grow as parents.

As I write this, I'm feeling our third baby moving in my belly. In two short weeks I will once again get to experience that sweet newborn smell, the sleepless nights, and around-the-clock feedings. I don't know yet what it's like to be a parent of three, but I know that there will be more love and less time.

Someone said to me the other day, "Just wait till they're all teenagers." These words reminded me of one of my favourite posts by blogger Katie Wetherbee, "Joy, or 'Just wait'?"[379] She points out that many people seem to have a chronic case of "just-wait-itis," which they pass on to new parents as a joke or as negative naysaying. "Just wait till she stops napping"; "just wait till he no longer kisses you goodbye." There's a good chance someone will say "just wait" to you, too. Don't take it to heart. There's so much to look forward to.

Just wait for his first real smile when his whole face lights up for you; wait to see the proud and surprised look on her face when she crawls for the first time; wait till he gives you his first sloppy kiss. There's so much to look forward to in the ever-important, challenging, beautiful, and special first year—and beyond. Just wait. Observe carefully, learn keenly, and love with all your heart. You've got this.

RECOMMENDED READING

For help creating a postpartum sanctuary:
- *The Fourth Trimester* by Kimberly Ann Johnson

To keep on your nightstand:
- *Becoming the Parent You Want to Be* by Laura Davis and Janis Keyser
- *The Baby Book* by William Sears, Martha Sears, Robert Sears, and James Sears

For inspiration and support:
- *Momma Zen* by Karen Maezen Miller
- *The Gifts of Imperfection* By Brené Brown
- *Raising Happiness* by Christine Carter

To broaden your cultural and societal perspectives on parenthood:
- *Our Babies, Ourselves* by Meredith F. Small
- *NurtureShock* by Po Bronson and Ashley Merryman
- *All Joy and No Fun* by Jennifer Senior

For ideas about feeding and cooking for babies and children:
- *Child of Mine: Feeding with Love and Good Sense* by Ellyn Satter
- *Wholefood for Children* by Jude Blereau

To learn more about child development:
- *The Whole-Brain Child* by Daniel J. Siegel and Tina Payne Bryson
- *The Philosophical Baby* by Alison Gopnik

To understand the science behind big parenting decisions and debates:
- *The Science of Mom* by Alice Callahan

To explore how to create a baby-friendly home:
- *Grow Healthy, Grow Happy* by Becky Cannon
- *Your Self-Confident Baby* by Magda Gerber and Allison Johnson

Looking ahead to the toddler years and beyond:
- *It's OK Not to Share* by Heather Shumaker
- *Siblings without Rivalry* by Adele Faber and Elaine Mazlish
- *Mindful Parenting* by Kristen Race
- *Punished by Rewards* by Alfie Kohn
- *No Bad Kids* by Janet Lansbury

ACKNOWLEDGEMENTS

The writing of this book spanned the full, messy, demanding, and beautiful years of my children's early childhood. Middle-of-the-night writing created space where my heart and mind could intersect fully. It could not have happened without the support and encouragement of others. I am so very grateful:

To my publishing team: Liz Trupin-Pulli, for believing in this project and for her advice; Jess Shulman, for looking at my manuscript with the sharp eye of an editor and the heart of a mother; Peter Bowerman, for help refining the title; and David Wogahn, Kerri Esten, and Manon Wogahn at AuthorImprints for the cover design, book interior layout, and for walking me through the publishing process.

To Dr. Luz Arbelaez for empowering me as a woman, and for bringing Ryan safely into the world.

To my friend Carrie Holt, for the forever-cherished support during and after our children's births.

To Bob and Donna Dunham, for being the best in-laws and grandparents one could hope for. I wish you were still here.

To my parents, Elena and Boris Epelbaum, and my grandparents, Alla Golodnova and Mark Epelbaum, for always being there for me and for showing me, back when I was little and to this day, what love, dedication, honour, and responsibility are. And to my little brother Dmitri Epelbaum, for reading early drafts and for being one of my very best friends.

To Leah, Tessa, and Ryan, for expanding my heart beyond what I thought possible and for being my reasons to grow and learn every day. And to Jason, for saying not only that I can write this book, but also that I must; for all the late-night discussions and edits; and for being my one. I love you.

BIBLIOGRAPHY

1. Bronfenbrenner U (1979) The ecology of human development. Harward University Press, Harward, MA, USA

2. Bronfenbrenner U (1992) Ecological systems theory. Pp. 187-249 in: Six theories of child development: revised formulations and current issues (ed. R. Vasta). Jessica Kingsley Publishers, London, England

3. Gopnik A (2016) The gardener and the carpenter: what the new science of child development tells us about the relationship between parents and children. Farrar, Strauss and Giroux, New York, NY, USA

4. Callahan A (2015) The Science of Mom: a research-based guide to your baby's first year. Johns Hopkins University Press, Baltimore, MD, USA

5. Nagy E (2011) The newborn infant: a missing stage in developmental psychology. Infant and Child Development 20(1): 3-19

6. Beebe B (2014) My journey in infant research and psychoanalysis: microanalysis, a social microscope. Psychoanalytic Psychology 31(1): 4-25

7. DeCasper A, Fifer W (1980) Of human bonding: newborns prefer their mothers' voices. Science 208(4448): 1174-1176

8. Kisilevsky BS et al (2003) Effects of experience on fetal voice recognition. Psychological Science 14(3): 220-224

9. Marshall J (2011) Infant neurosensory development: considerations for infant child care. Early Childhood Education Journal 39(3): 175-181

10. Moon C, Cooper RP, Fifer WP (1993) Two-day-olds prefer their native language. Infant Behavior and Development 16(4): 495-500

11. DeCasper AJ, Lecanuet J-P, Busnel M-C, Granier-Deferre C, Maugeais R. (1994) Fetal reactions to recurrent maternal speech. Infant Behavior and Development 17(2): 159-164

12. Slater A (2002) Visual perception in the newborn infant: issues and debates. Intellectica 34: 57-76

13. Mondloch CJ et al (1999) Face perception during early infancy. Psychological Science 10(5): 419-422

14. Sai FZ (2005) The role of the mother's voice in developing mother's face preference: evidence for intermodal perception at birth. Infant and Child Development 14(1): 29-50

15. Farroni T et al (2002) Eye contact detection in humans from birth. Proceedings of the National Academy of Sciences 99(14): 9602-9605

16. White-Traut RC et al (2009) Salivary cortisol and behavioral state responses of healthy newborn infants to tactile-only and multisensory interventions. Journal of Obstetric, Gynecologic and Neonatal Nursing 38(1): 22-34

17. Mennella JA (1995) Mother's milk: a medium for early flavor experiences. Journal of Human Lactation 11(1): 39-45

18. Schaal B, Marlier L, Soussignan R (2000) Human foetuses learn odours from their pregnant mother's diet. Chemical Senses 25(6): 729-737

19. Klaus M (1998) Mother and infant: early emotional ties. Pediatrics 102(Supplement E1): 1244-1246

20. Rosenblum KL, Dayton CJ, Muzik M (2009) Infant social and emotional development: emerging competence in a relational context. Pp. 80-103 in: Handbook of infant mental health, 3rd ed. (ed. C. H. Zeanah Jr.). The Guilford Press, New York, NY, USA

21. Porges SW (1992) Vagal tone: a physiologic marker of stress vulnerability. Pediatrics 90(3): 498-504

22. Feldman R, Eidelman AI (2009) Biological and environmental initial conditions shape the trajectories of cognitive and social-emotional development across the first years of life. Developmental Science 12(1): 194-200

23. Thomas A, Chess S (1977) Temperament and development. Brunner/Mazel, Oxford, England.

24. Rothbart MK (1981) Measurement of temperament in infancy. Child Development 52(2): 569-578

25. Kagan J (1997) Temperament and the reactions to unfamiliarity. Child Development 68(1): 139-143

26. Leerkes EM, Blankson AN, O'Brien M (2009) Differential effects of maternal sensitivity to infant distress and nondistress on social-emotional functioning. Child Development 80(3): 762-775

27. Wolke D, Bilgin A, Samara M (2017) Systematic review and meta-analysis: fussing and crying durations and prevalence of colic in infants. The Journal of Pediatrics 185: 55-61. e4

28. Van Ijzendoorn MH, Hubbard FOA (2000) Are infant crying and maternal responsiveness during the first year related to infant-mother attachment at 15 months? Attachment and Human Development 2(3): 371-391

29. Wessel MA et al (1954) Paroxysmal fussing in infancy, sometimes called "colic" Pediatrics 14(5): 421-435

30. White BP et al (2000) Behavioral and physiological responsivity, sleep, and patterns of daily cortisol production in infants with and without colic. Child Development 71(4): 862-877

31. Stifter CA, Bono MA (1998) The effect of infant colic on maternal self-perceptions and mother-infant attachment. Child: Care, Health and Development 24(5): 339-351

32. Dubois NE, Gregory KE (2016) Characterizing the intestinal microbiome in infantile colic: findings based on an integrative review of the literature. Biological Research For Nursing 18(3): 307-315

33. Sung V et al (2018) *Lactobacillus reuteri* to treat infant colic: a meta-analysis. Pediatrics 141(1): e20171811

34. Ong TG et al (2019) Probiotics to prevent infantile colic. Cochrane Database of Systematic Reviews 3(3): Cd012473

35. Bornstein MH et al (2017) Neurobiology of culturally common maternal responses to infant cry. Proceedings of the National Academy of Sciences 114(45): E9465-E73

36. Ainsworth MS, Bowlby J (1991) An ethological approach to personality development. American Psychologist 46(4): 333-341

37. Bretherton 1 (1992) The origins of attachment theory: John Bowlby and Mary Ainsworth. Developmental Psychology 28(5): 759-775

38. Larkin F et al (2019) Proof of concept of a smartphone app to support delivery of an intervention to facilitate mothers' mind-mindedness. PLoS One 14(8): e0220948

39. Meins E et al (2011). Mother- versus infant-centered correlates of maternal mind-mindedness in the first year of life. Infancy 16(2): 137-165

40. Koren-Karie N et al (2002) Mothers' insightfulness regarding their infants' internal experience: relations with maternal sensitivity and infant attachment. Developmental Psychology 38(4): 534-542

41. Zeegers MAJ et al (2018) Mothers' and fathers' mind-mindedness influences physiological emotion regulation of infants across the first year of life. Developmental Science 21(6): e12689

42. Meins E et al (2006) Mind-mindedness in children: individual differences in internal-state talk in middle childhood. British Journal of Developmental Psychology 24(1): 181-196

43. Farrow C, Blissett J (2014) Maternal mind-mindedness during infancy, general parenting sensitivity and observed child feeding behavior: a longitudinal study. Attachment and Human Development 16(3): 230-241

44. Davis KF, Parker KP, Montgomery GL (2004) Sleep in infants and young children. Part one: normal sleep. Journal of Pediatric Health Care 18(2): 65-71

45. Rauchs G et al (2008) Sleep modulates the neural substrates of both spatial and contextual memory consolidation. PLoS One 3(8): e2949

46. Horváth K et al (2018) Memory in 3-month-old infants benefits from a short nap. Developmental Science 21(3): e12587

47. Tomalski P et al (2017) Chaotic home environment is associated with reduced infant processing speed under high task demands. Infant Behavior and Development 48: 124-133

48. Marcus GF et al (1999) Rule learning by seven-month-old infants. Science 283(5398): 77-80

49. Needham A, Baillargeon R (1993) Intuitions about support in 4.5-month-old infants. Cognition 47(2): 121-148

50. Maurer D, Lewis TL (1979) A physiological explanation of infants' early visual development. Canadian Journal of Psychology 33(4): 232-252

51. PrabhuDas M et al (2011) Challenges in infant immunity: implications for responses to infection and vaccines. Nature Immunology 12(3): 189-194

52. Hotelling BA (2004) Newborn capabilities: parent teaching is a necessity. Journal of Perinatal Education 13(4): 43-49

53. Sytsma SE, Kelley ML, Wymer JH (2001) Development and initial validation of the child routines inventory. Journal of Psychopathology and Behavioral Assessment 23(4): 241-251

54. Fantasia V et al (2016) Not just being lifted: infants are sensitive to delay during a pick-up routine. Frontiers in Psychology 6: 2065

55. Armstrong KL, Quinn RA, Dadds MR (1994) The sleep patterns of normal children. Medical Journal of Australia 161(3): 202-205

56. Mindell JA et al (1994) Pediatricians and sleep disorders: training and practice. Pediatrics 94(2 Pt 1): 194-200

57. Owens JA (2001) The practice of pediatric sleep medicine: results of a community survey. Pediatrics 108(3): E51

58. Boreman CD et al (2007) Resident training in developmental/behavioral pediatrics: where do we stand? Clinical Pediatrics 46(2): 135-145

59. Ramos KD, Youngclarke DM (2006) Parenting advice books about child sleep: cosleeping and crying it out. Sleep 29(12): 1616-1623

60. Hiscock H, Fisher J (2015) Sleeping like a baby? Infant sleep: impact on caregivers and current controversies. Journal of Paediatrics and Child Health 51(4): 361-364

61. Sadeh A (2001) Sleeping Like a Baby: a sensitive and sensible approach to solving your child's sleep problems. Yale University Press, New Haven, CT, USA

62. Turgeon H, Wright J (2014) The Happy Sleeper: the science-backed guide to helping your baby get a good night's sleep - newborn to school age. he Penguin Group, New York, NY, USA

63. Ednick M et al (2009) A review of the effects of sleep during the first year of life on cognitive, psychomotor, and temperament development. Sleep 32(11): 1449-1458

64. Dahl RE (1998) The development and disorders of sleep. Advances in Pediatrics 45: 73-90

65. Marks GA et al (1995) A functional role for REM sleep in brain maturation. Behavioural Brain Research 69(1): 1-11

66. Walker MP, van der Helm E (2009) Overnight therapy? The role of sleep in emotional brain processing. Psychological Bulletin 135(5): 731-748

67. Walker MP, Stickgold R (2010) Overnight alchemy: sleep-dependent memory evolution. Nature Reviews Neuroscience 11(3): 218

68. Diekelmann S, Born J (2010) The memory function of sleep. Nature Reviews Neuroscience 11(2): 114-126

69. Scher A (2005) Infant sleep at 10 months of age as a window to cognitive development. Early Human Development 81(3): 289-292

70. Sadeh A et al (2015) Infant sleep predicts attention regulation and behavior problems at 3—4 years of age. Developmental Neuropsychology 40(3): 122-137

71. Takahashi Y, Kipnis DM, Daughaday WH (1968) Growth hormone secretion during sleep. The Journal of Clinical Investigation 47(9): 2079-2090

72. Tikotzky et al (2010) Sleep and physical growth in infants during the first 6 months. Journal of Sleep Research 19(1 Pt 1): 103-110

73. Bryant PA, Trinder J, Curtis N (2004) Sick and tired: does sleep have a vital role in the immune system? Nature Reviews Immunology 4(6): 457-467

74. Aldabal L, Bahammam AS (2011) Metabolic, endocrine, and immune consequences of sleep deprivation. The Open Respiratory Medicine Journal 5: 31-43

75. Bordeleau S, Bernier A, Carrier J (2012) Maternal sensitivity and children's behavior problems: examining the moderating role of infant sleep duration. Journal of Clinical Child and Adolescent Psychology 41(4): 471-481

76. Bernier A et al (2014) My mother is sensitive, but I am too tired to know: infant sleep as a moderator of prospective relations between maternal sensitivity and infant outcomes. Infant Behavior and Development 37(4): 682-694

77. Dijk D-J, Czeisler CA (1994) Paradoxical timing of the circadian rhythm of sleep propensity serves to consolidate sleep and wakefulness in humans. Neuroscience Letters 166(1): 63-68

78. Mirmiran M, Maas YGH, Ariagno RL (2003) Development of fetal and neonatal sleep and circadian rhythms. Sleep Medicine Reviews 7(4): 321-334

79. McGraw K et al (1999) The development of circadian rhythms in a human infant. Sleep 22(3): 303-310

80. Coons S, Guilleminault C (1982) Development of sleep-wake patterns and non-rapid eye movement sleep stages during the first six months of life in normal infants. Pediatrics 69(6): 793-798

81. Anders TF, Halpern LF, Hua J (1992) Sleeping through the night: a developmental perspective. Pediatrics 90(4): 554-560

82. Henderson JMT, France KG, Blampied NM (2011) The consolidation of infants' nocturnal sleep across the first year of life. Sleep Medicine Reviews 15(4): 211-220

83. Burnham MM et al (2002) Nighttime sleep-wake patterns and self-soothing from birth to one year of age: a longitudinal intervention study. Journal of Child Psychology and Psychiatry 43(6): 713-725

84. Kennaway DJ, Goble FC, Stamp GE (1996) Factors influencing the development of melatonin rhythmicity in humans. The Journal of Clinical Endocrinology and Metabolism 81(4): 1525-1532

85. Sadeh A (1997) Sleep and melatonin in infants: a preliminary study. Sleep 20(3): 185-191

86. de Weerd AW, van den Bossche RAS (2003) The development of sleep during the first months of life. Sleep Medicine Reviews 7(2): 179-191

87. Goodlin-Jones BL et al (2001) Night waking, sleep-wake organization, and self-soothing in the first year of life. Journal of Developmental and Behavioral Pediatrics 22(4): 226-233

88. Jenni O, Carskadon M (2000) Normal human sleep at different ages: infants to adolescents. Pp 11-19 in: SRS Basics of Sleep Guide, Sleep Research Society, Westchester, IL, USA

89. Ferber R (2006) Solve your child's sleep problems: new, revised, and expanded edition. Touchstone, New York, NY, USA

90. Adair RH, Bauchner H (1993) Sleep problems in childhood. Current Problems in Pediatrics 23(4): 147-170

91. Moore T, Ucko LE (1957) Night waking in early infancy. Archives of Disease in Childhood 32(164): 333-342

92. Anders TF (1979) Night-waking in infants during the first year of life. Pediatrics 63(6): 860-864

93. Ferber R, Boyle M (1983) Sleeplessness in infants and toddlers: sleep initiation difficulty masquerading as a sleep maintenance insomnia. Sleep Research 12: 240-243

94. Anders TF, Keener M (1985) Developmental course of nighttime sleep-wake patterns in full-term and premature infants during the first year of life. Sleep 8(3): 173-192

95. Keener MA, Zeanah CH, Anders TF (1988) Infant temperament, sleep organization, and nighttime parental interventions. Pediatrics 81(6): 762-771

96. Iglowstein I et al (2003) Sleep duration from infancy to adolescence: reference values and generational trends. Pediatrics 111(2): 302-307

97. Mindell JA et al (2010) Cross-cultural differences in infant and toddler sleep. Sleep Medicine 11(3): 274-280

98. Sadeh A et al (2009) Sleep and sleep ecology in the first 3 years: a web-based study. Journal of Sleep Research 18(1): 60-73

99. Fisher A et al (2012) Genetic and environmental influences on infant sleep. Pediatrics 129(6): 1091-1096

100. Tikotzky L, Sadeh A (2009) Maternal sleep-related cognitions and infant sleep: a longitudinal study from pregnancy through the 1st year. Child Development 80(3): 860-874

101. Brescianini S et al (2011) Genetic and environmental factors shape infant sleep patterns: a study of 18-month-old twins. Pediatrics 127(5): e1296-e1302

102. Teti DM et al (2010) Maternal emotional availability at bedtime predicts infant sleep quality. Journal of Family Psychology 24(3): 307-315

103. Gilbert R et al (2005) Infant sleeping position and the sudden infant death syndrome: systematic review of observational studies and historical review of recommendations from 1940 to 2002. International Journal of Epidemiology 34(4): 874-887

104. Kahn A et al (1993) Prone or supine body position and sleep characteristics in infants. Pediatrics 91(6): 1112-1115

105. Franco P et al (2010) Arousal from sleep mechanisms in infants. Sleep Medicine 11(7): 603-614

106. McKenna JJ (1995) The potential benefits of infant—parent co-sleeping in relation to SIDS prevention: overview and critique of epidemiological bed sharing studies. Pp 256-265 in: Sudden infant death syndrome: New trends in the nineties (ed Rognum TO), Scandinavian University Press, Oslo, Norway

107. Ward TCS (2015) Reasons for mother—infant bed-sharing: a systematic narrative synthesis of the literature and implications for future research. Maternal and Child Health Journal 19(3): 675-690

108. McKenna JJ, McDade T (2005) Why babies should never sleep alone: a review of the co-sleeping controversy in relation to SIDS, bedsharing and breast feeding. Paediatric Respiratory Reviews 6(2): 134-152

109. Blair PS et al (2014) Bed-sharing in the absence of hazardous circumstances: is there a risk of sudden infant death syndrome? An analysis from two case-control studies conducted in the UK. PLoS One 9(9): e107799

110. Carpenter R et al (2013) Bed sharing when parents do not smoke: is there a risk of SIDS? An individual level analysis of five major case—control studies. BMJ open 3(5): e002299

111. American Academy of Pediatrics (2016) SIDS and other sleep-related infant deaths: updated 2016 recommendations for a safe infant sleeping environment. Pediatrics 138(5): e20162938

112. Mosko S, Richard C, McKenna J (1997) Infant arousals during mother-infant bed sharing: implications for infant sleep and sudden infant death syndrome research. Pediatrics 100(5): 841-849

113. Touchette É et al (2005) Factors associated with fragmented sleep at night across early childhood. Archives of Pediatrics and Adolescent Medicine 159(3): 242-249

114. Jenni OG et al (2005) A longitudinal study of bed sharing and sleep problems among Swiss children in the first 10 years of life. Pediatrics 115(Supplement 1): 233-240

115. Mao A et al (2004) A comparison of the sleep—wake patterns of cosleeping and solitary-sleeping infants. Child Psychiatry and Human Development 35(2): 95-105

116. Baddock SA et al (2006) Differences in infant and parent behaviors during routine bed sharing compared with cot sleeping in the home setting. Pediatrics 117(5): 1599-1607

117. Volkovich E et al (2015) Sleep patterns of co-sleeping and solitary sleeping infants and mothers: a longitudinal study. Sleep Medicine 16(11): 1305-1312

118. Morelli GA et al (1992) Cultural variation in infants' sleeping arrangements: questions of independence. Developmental Psychology 28(4): 604-613

119. Ramos KD (2003) Intentional versus reactive cosleeping. Sleep Research Online 5:141-147

120. DeLeon CW, Karraker KH (2007) Intrinsic and extrinsic factors associated with night waking in 9-month-old infants. Infant behavior and Development 30(4): 596-605

121. Weissbluth M (2015) Healthy sleep habits, happy child: a step-by-step program for a good night's sleep (4th ed). Ballantine Books, USA

122. Jenni OG, Deboer T, Achermann P (2006) Development of the 24-h rest-activity pattern in human infants. Infant Behavior and Development 29(2): 143-152

123. Cespedes EM et al (2014) Television viewing, bedroom television, and sleep duration from infancy to mid-childhood. Pediatrics 133(5): e1163-e1171

124. Cheung CHM et al (2017) Daily touchscreen use in infants and toddlers is associated with reduced sleep and delayed sleep onset. Scientific Reports 7(1): 46104

125. Engler AC et al (2012) Breastfeeding may improve nocturnal sleep and reduce infantile colic: potential role of breast milk melatonin. European Journal of Pediatrics 171(4): 729-732

126. Illnerova H, Buresova M, Presl J (1993) Melatonin rhythm in human milk. The Journal of Clinical Endocrinology and Metabolism 77(3): 838-841

127. France KG, Blampied NM (1999) Infant sleep disturbance: description of a problem behaviour process. Sleep Medicine Reviews 3(4): 265-280

128. Thoman EB (1990) Sleeping and waking states in infants: a functional perspective. Neuroscience and Biobehavioral Reviews 14(1): 93-107

129. Latz S, Wolf AW, Lozoff B (1999) Cosleeping in context: sleep practices and problems in young children in Japan and the United States. Archives of Pediatrics and Adolescent Medicine 153(4): 339-346

130. Adair R et al (1991) Night waking during infancy: role of parental presence at bedtime. Pediatrics 87(4): 500-504

131. Scher A, Asher R (2004) Is attachment security related to sleep—wake regulation? Mothers' reports and objective sleep recordings. Infant Behavior and Development 27(3): 288-302

132. Stamm J, Spencer P (2007) Bright from the start: the simple, science-backed way to nurture your child's developing mind, from birth to age 3. Penguin, USA

133. Skuladottir A, Thome M, Ramel A (2005) Improving day and night sleep problems in infants by changing day time sleep rhythm: a single group before and after study. International Journal of Nursing Studies 42(8): 843-850

134. Pinilla T, Birch LL (1993) Help me make it through the night: behavioral entrainment of breast-fed infants' sleep patterns. Pediatrics 91(2): 436-444

135. Brown A, Harries V (2015) Infant sleep and night feeding patterns during later infancy: association with breastfeeding frequency, daytime complementary food intake, and infant weight. Breastfeeding Medicine 10(5): 246-252

136. Macknin ML et al (2000) Symptoms associated with infant teething: a prospective study. Pediatrics 105(4): 747-752

137. Owais A, Zawaideh F, Bataineh O (2010) Challenging parents' myths regarding their children's teething. International Journal of Dental Hygiene 8(1): 28-34

138. Wake M, Hesketh K, Lucas J (2000) Teething and tooth eruption in infants: a cohort study. Pediatrics 106(6): 1374-1379

139. Markman L (2009) Teething: facts and fiction. Pediatrics in Review 30(8): e59-e64

140. Ramos-Jorge J et al (2011) Prospective longitudinal study of signs and symptoms associated with primary tooth eruption. Pediatrics 128(3): 471-476

141. Memarpour M, Soltanimehr E, Eskandarian T (2015) Signs and symptoms associated with primary tooth eruption: a clinical trial of nonpharmacological remedies. BMC Oral Health 15(88)

142. Williams GD et al (2011) Salicylate intoxication from teething gel in infancy. The Medical Journal of Australia 194(3): 146-148

143. Liaw R et al (2019) Infant deaths in sitting devices. Pediatrics 144(1): e20182576

144. Public Health Agency of Canada (2014) Safe sleep for your baby. Health Canada, Ottawa, ON, Canada

145. Hugh SC et al (2014) Infant sleep machines and hazardous sound pressure levels. Pediatrics 133(4): 677-681

146. Kirjavainen J et al (2001) Infants with colic have a normal sleep structure at 2 and 7 months of age. The Journal of Pediatrics 138(2): 218-223

147. Miller KM (2007) Momma Zen: walking the crooked path of motherhood. Shambhala Publications, Boulder, CO, USA

148. Hauck FR et al (2003) Sleep environment and the risk of sudden infant death syndrome in an urban population: the Chicago Infant Mortality Study. Pediatrics 111(Supplement 1): 1207-1214

149. Schwartz C et al (2011) Development of healthy eating habits early in life. Review of recent evidence and selected guidelines. Appetite 57(3): 796-807

150. Savage JS, Fisher JO, Birch LL (2007) Parental influence on eating behavior: conception to adolescence. The Journal of Law, Medicine and Ethics 35(1): 22-34

151. Victora CG et al. (2016) Breastfeeding in the 21st century: epidemiology, mechanisms, and lifelong effect. The Lancet 387(10017): 475-490

152. McDade TW (2003) Life history theory and the immune system: steps toward a human ecological immunology. American Journal of Physical Anthropology 122(S37): 100-125

153. Gura T (2014) Nature's first functional food. Science 345(6198): 747-749

154. Underwood MA (2013) Human milk for the premature infant. Pediatric Clinics 60(1): 189-207

155. Patel AL, Kim JH (2018) Human milk and necrotizing enterocolitis. Seminars in Pediatric Surgery 27(1): 34-38

156. Pabst H, Spady D (1990) Effect of breast-feeding on antibody response to conjugate vaccine. The Lancet 336(8710): 269-270

157. Guilbert TW et al (2007) Effect of breastfeeding on lung function in childhood and modulation by maternal asthma and atopy. American Journal of Respiratory and Critical Care Medicine 176(9): 843-848

158. Mueller NT et al (2015) The infant microbiome development: mom matters. Trends in Molecular Medicine 21(2): 109-117

159. Baquero F, Nombela C (2012) The microbiome as a human organ. Clinical Microbiology and Infection 18: 2-4

160. Perez-Muñoz ME et al (2017) A critical assessment of the "sterile womb" and "in utero colonization" hypotheses: implications for research on the pioneer infant microbiome. Microbiome 5: 48

161. Albenberg LG, Wu GD (2014) Diet and the intestinal microbiome: associations, functions, and implications for health and disease. Gastroenterology 146(6): 1564-1572

162. Hausner H et al (2010) Breastfeeding facilitates acceptance of a novel dietary flavour compound. Clinical Nutrition 29(1): 141-148

163. Harris G, Coulthard H (2016) Early eating behaviours and food acceptance revisited: breastfeeding and introduction of complementary foods as predictive of food acceptance. Current Obesity Reports 5(1): 113-120

164. Morley R et al (1988) Mother's choice to provide breast milk and developmental outcome. Archives of Disease in Childhood 63(11): 1382-1385

165. Kramer MS, et al (2008) Breastfeeding and child cognitive development: new evidence from a large randomized trial. Archives of General Psychiatry 65(5): 578-584

166. Deoni SC et al (2013) Breastfeeding and early white matter development: a cross-sectional study. Neuroimage 82: 77-86

167. Martens PJ (2012) What do Kramer's Baby-Friendly Hospital Initiative PROBIT studies tell us? A review of a decade of research. Journal of Human Lactation 28(3): 335-342

168. Luby JL et al (2016) Breastfeeding and childhood IQ: the mediating role of gray matter volume. Journal of the American Academy of Child and Adolescent Psychiatry 55(5): 367-375

169. Eidelman AI (2013) Breastfeeding and cognitive development: is there an association? Jornal de Pediatria 89(4): 327-329

170. Der G, Batty GD, Deary IJ (2006) Effect of breast feeding on intelligence in children: prospective study, sibling pairs analysis, and meta-analysis. BMJ 333(7575): 945

171. Evenhouse E, Reilly S (2005) Improved estimates of the benefits of breastfeeding using sibling comparisons to reduce selection bias. Health Services Research 40(6 pt 1): 1781-1802

172. Colen CG, Ramey DM (2014) Is breast truly best? Estimating the effects of breastfeeding on long-term child health and wellbeing in the United States using sibling comparisons. Social Science and Medicine 109: 55-65

173. Montgomery SM, Ehlin A, Sacker A (2006) Breast feeding and resilience against psychosocial stress. Archives of Disease in Childhood 91(12): 990-994

174. Oddy WH et al (2010) The long-term effects of breastfeeding on child and adolescent mental health: a pregnancy cohort study followed for 14 years. The Journal of Pediatrics 156(4): 568-574

175. Lee S, Kelleher SL (2016) Biological underpinnings of breastfeeding challenges: the role of genetics, diet, and environment on lactation physiology. American Journal of Physiology-Endocrinology and Metabolism 311(2): E405-E422

176. Colin WB, Scott JA (2002) Breastfeeding: reasons for starting, reasons for stopping and problems along the way. Breastfeeding Review 10(2): 13-19

177. Kent JC (2007) How breastfeeding works. Journal of Midwifery and Women's Health 52(6): 564-570

178. Amir LH (2014) Managing common breastfeeding problems in the community. BMJ 348: g2954

179. Buck ML et al (2014) Nipple pain, damage, and vasospasm in the first 8 weeks postpartum. Breastfeeding Medicine 9(2): 56-62

180. Gribble KD (2008) Long-term breastfeeding; changing attitudes and overcoming challenges. Breastfeeding Review 16(1): 5-15

181. Edmunds J, Miles S, Fulbrook P (2011) Tongue-tie and breastfeeding: a review of the literature. Breastfeeding Review 19(1): 19-26

182. Segal LM et al (2007) Prevalence, diagnosis, and treatment of ankyloglossia. Methodologic Review. Canadian Family Physician 53(6): 1027-1033

183. Berry J, Griffiths M, Westcott C (2012) A double-blind, randomized, controlled trial of tongue-tie division and its immediate effect on breastfeeding. Breastfeeding Medicine 7(3): 189-193

184. Hogan M, Westcott C, Griffiths M (2005) Randomized, controlled trial of division of tongue-tie in infants with feeding problems. Journal of Paediatrics and Child Health 41: 246-250

185. Dewey KG, Lönnerdal B (1986) Infant self-regulation of breast milk intake. Acta Paediatrica 75(6): 893-898

186. Kent JC et al (2006) Volume and frequency of breastfeedings and fat content of breast milk throughout the day. Pediatrics 117(3): e387-e395

187. Li R, Fein SB, Grummer-Strawn LM (2010) Do infants fed from bottles lack self-regulation of milk intake compared with directly breastfed infants? Pediatrics 125(6): e1386-e1393

188. Brown A, Lee M (2012) Breastfeeding during the first year promotes satiety responsiveness in children aged 18—24 months. Pediatric Obesity 7(5): 382-390

189. Innis SM (2008) Dietary omega 3 fatty acids and the developing brain. Brain Research 1237: 35-43

190. Jenik AG et al (2009) Does the recommendation to use a pacifier influence the prevalence of breastfeeding? The Journal of Pediatrics 155(3): 350-354.e1

191. Nelson AM (2012) A comprehensive review of evidence and current recommendations related to pacifier usage. Journal of Pediatric Nursing 27(6): 690-699

192. Silveira LM et al (2013) Influence of breastfeeding on children's oral skills. Revista de Saúde Pública 47(1): 37-43

193. McCann JC, Ames BN (2005) Is docosahexaenoic acid, an n-3 long-chain polyunsaturated fatty acid, required for development of normal brain function? An overview of evidence from cognitive and behavioral tests in humans and animals. The American Journal of Clinical Nutrition 82(2): 281-95

194. Delplanque B et al (2015) Lipid quality in infant nutrition: current knowledge and future opportunities. Journal of Pediatric Gastroenterology and Nutrition 61(1): 8-17

195. Veereman-Wauters G et al (2011) Physiological and bifidogenic effects of prebiotic supplements in infant formulae. Journal of Pediatric Gastroenterology and Nutrition 52(6): 763-771

196. Krebs NF et al (2013) Effects of different complementary feeding regimens on iron status and enteric microbiota in breastfed infants. The Journal of Pediatrics 163(2): 416-423.e4

197. Carruth BR, Skinner JD (2002) Feeding behaviors and other motor development in healthy children (2—24 Months). Journal of the American College of Nutrition 21(2): 88-96

198. Skinner JD et al (1998) Mealtime communication patterns of infants from 2 to 24 months of age. Journal of Nutrition Education 30(1): 8-16

199. Davis CM (1928) Self-selection of diet by newly weaned infants: an experimental study. American Journal of Diseases of Children 36(4): 651-679

200. Davis CM (1939) Results of self-selection of diets by young children. Canadian Medical Association Journal 41(3): 257-261

201. Cohen RJ et al (1994) Effects of age of introduction of complementary foods on infant breast milk intake, total energy intake, and growth: a randomised intervention study in Honduras. The Lancet 344(8918): 288-293

202. Farrow C, Blissett J (2006) Does maternal control during feeding moderate early infant weight gain? Pediatrics 118(2): e293-e298

203. Black MM, Aboud FE (2011) Responsive feeding is embedded in a theoretical framework of responsive parenting. The Journal of Nutrition 141(3): 490-494

204. Satter E (2000) Child of Mine: feeding with love and good sense (3rd edition). Bull Publishing Company, Boulder, CO, USA

205. Butte N et al (2004) The Start Healthy feeding guidelines for infants and toddlers. Journal of the American Dietetic Association 104(3): 442-454

206. Rapley G et al (2015) Baby-Led Weaning: a new frontier? ICAN: Infant, Child, and Adolescent Nutrition 7(2): 77-85

207. Cameron SL, Taylor RW, Heath A-LM (2013) Parent-led or baby-led? Associations between complementary feeding practices and health-related behaviours in a survey of New Zealand families. BMJ Open 3(12): e003946

208. Fangupo LJ et al (2016) A baby-led approach to eating solids and risk of choking. Pediatrics 138(4): e20160772

209. Williams Erickson L et al (2018) Impact of a modified version of baby-led weaning on infant food and nutrient intakes: the BLISS randomized controlled trial. Nutrients 10(6): 740

210. Daniels L et al (2018) Impact of a modified version of baby-led weaning on iron intake and status: a randomised controlled trial. BMJ Open 8(6): e019036

211. Carruth BR et al (2004) Prevalence of picky eaters among infants and toddlers and their caregivers' decisions about offering a new food. Journal of the American Dietetic Association 104: 57-64

212. Nicklaus S (2011) Children's acceptance of new foods at weaning. Role of practices of weaning and of food sensory properties. Appetite 57(3): 812-825

213. Maier A et al (2007) Effects of repeated exposure on acceptance of initially disliked vegetables in 7-month old infants. Food Quality and Preference 18(8): 1023-1032

214. Gerrish CJ, Mennella JA (2001) Flavor variety enhances food acceptance in formula-fed infants. The American Journal of Clinical Nutrition 73(6): 1080-1085

215. Mennella JA et al (2008) Variety is the spice of life: strategies for promoting fruit and vegetable acceptance during infancy. Physiology and Behavior 94(1): 29-38

216. Dewey KG (2013) The challenge of meeting nutrient needs of infants and young children during the period of complementary feeding: an evolutionary perspective. The Journal of Nutrition 143(12): 2050-2054

217. American Academy of Pediatrics (2018) Red Book: 2018-2021 report of the committee on infectious diseases (eds Kimberlin DW, Barnett ED, Lynfield R, Sawyer MH). Itasca, IL, USA

218. Roess AA et al (2018) Food consumption patterns of infants and toddlers: findings from the Feeding Infants and Toddlers Study (FITS) 2016. The Journal of Nutrition 148(suppl 3): 1525S-1535S

219. Wagner CL, Greer FR (2008) Prevention of rickets and vitamin D deficiency in infants, children, and adolescents. Pediatrics 122(5): 1142-1152

220. Dube K et al (2010) Iron intake and iron status in breastfed infants during the first year of life. Clinical Nutrition 29(6): 773-778

221. Grimes CA et al (2015) Food sources of total energy and nutrients among U.S. infants and toddlers: National Health and Nutrition Examination Survey 2005—2012. Nutrients 7(8): 6797-6836

222. Davidsson L (2003) Approaches to improve iron bioavailability from complementary foods. The Journal of Nutrition 133(5): 1560S-1562S

223. Hirsch J (2018) Heavy metals in baby food: what you need to know. Consumer Reports. https://www.consumerreports.org/food-safety/heavy-metals-in-baby-food/ (accessed on June 20, 2021)

224. Fikiru Dasa TA (2018) Factors affecting iron absorption and mitigation mechanisms: a review. International Journal of Agricultural Science and Food Technology 4(1): 24-30

225. Ziegler EE (2011) Consumption of cow's milk as a cause of iron deficiency in infants and toddlers. Nutrition Reviews 69(suppl 1): S37-S42

226. U.S. Department of Agriculture (2020) FoodData Central. https://fdc.nal.usda.gov/ (accessed on June 20, 2021)

227. Dewey K (2003) Guiding principles for complementary feeding of the breastfed child. Pan American Health Organization, World Health Organization, Washington, DC, USA

228. World Health Organization (2005) Guiding principles for feeding non-breastfed children 6-24 months of age. Geneva, Switzerland

229. Karsten HD et al (2010) Vitamins A, E and fatty acid composition of the eggs of caged hens and pastured hens. Renewable Agriculture and Food Systems 25(1): 45-54

230. Grimshaw KEC et al (2014) Diet and food allergy development during infancy: birth cohort study findings using prospective food diary data. Journal of Allergy and Clinical Immunology 133(2): 511-519

231. García AL et al (2013) Nutritional content of infant commercial weaning foods in the UK. Archives of Disease in Childhood 98(10): 793-797

232. Moore ER et al (2016) Early skin-to-skin contact for mothers and their healthy newborn infants. Cochrane Database of Systematic Reviews 2016, Issue 11

233. Lavelli M, Poli M (1998) Early mother-infant interaction during breast- and bottle-feeding. Infant Behavior and Development 21(4): 667-683

234. Ricke LA et al (2005) Newborn tongue-tie: prevalence and effect on breast-feeding. The Journal of the American Board of Family Practice 18(1): 1-7

235. Fernando N, Potock M (2015) Raising a healthy, happy eater: a stage-by-stage guide to setting your child on the path to adventurous eating. The Experiment, New York, NY, USA

236. Ventura AK, Beauchamp GK, Mennella JA (2012) Infant regulation of intake: the effect of free glutamate content in infant formulas. The American Journal of Clinical Nutrition 95(4): 875-881

237. Shloim N et al (2017) Looking for cues—infant communication of hunger and satiation during milk feeding. Appetite 108: 74-82

238. Ventura AK, Inamdar LB, Mennella JA (2015) Consistency in infants' behavioural signalling of satiation during bottle-feeding. Pediatric Obesity 10(3): 180-187

239. Ventura AK, Mennella JA (2017) An experimental approach to study individual differences in infants' intake and satiation behaviors during bottle-feeding. Childhood Obesity 13(1): 44-52

240. Chapin MM et al (2013) Nonfatal choking on food among children 14 years or younger in the United States, 2001—2009. Pediatrics 132(2): 275-281

241. Blereau J (2019) Wholefood for children: nourishing young children with whole and organic foods (2nd edition). Murdoch Books, London, UK

242. Huggins K, Petok E, Mireles O (2000) Markers of lactation insufficiency: a study of 34 mothers. Current Issues in Clinical Lactation 1: 25-35

243. Moore GA, Calkins SD (2004) Infants' vagal regulation in the still-face paradigm is related to dyadic coordination of mother-infant interaction. Developmental Psychology 40(6): 1068-1080

244. Adamson LB, Frick JE (2003) The Still Face: a history of a shared experimental paradigm. Infancy 4(4): 451-473

245. Reddy V (2015) Joining Intentions in Infancy. Journal of Consciousness Studies 22(1-2): 24-44

246. Mandel DR, Jusczyk PW, Pisoni DB (1995) Infants' recognition of the sound patterns of their own names. Psychological Science 6(5): 314-317

247. Lloyd-Fox S et al (2015) Are you talking to me? Neural activations in 6-month-old infants in response to being addressed during natural interactions. Cortex 70: 35-48

248. Erickson LC, Newman RS (2017) Influences of background noise on infants and children. Current Directions in Psychological Science 26(5): 451-457

249. Golinkoff RM et al (2015) (Baby) talk to me: the social context of infant-directed speech and its effects on early language acquisition. Current Directions in Psychological Science 24(5): 339-344

250. Bergelson E, Aslin RN (2017) Nature and origins of the lexicon in 6-mo-olds. Proceedings of the National Academy of Sciences 114(49): 12916-12921

251. Hamlin JK, Wynn K, Bloom P (2007) Social evaluation by preverbal infants. Nature 450: 557-559

252. Sorce JF et al (1985) Maternal emotional signaling: its effect on the visual cliff behavior of 1-year-olds. Developmental Psychology 21(1): 195-200

253. Erikson EH (1959) Identity and the life cycle: selected papers. International Universities Press, Oxford, UK

254. Ainsworth MDS, Bell SM, Stayton DF (1974) Infant-mother attachment and social development: Socialization as a product of reciprocal responsiveness to signals. Pp 99-135 in: The integration of a child into a social world (ed Richards MPM). Cambridge University Press, New York, NY, USA

255. Bell SM, Ainsworth MD (1972) Infant crying and maternal responsiveness. Child Development 43(4): 1171-119.

256. Landry SH, Smith KE, Swank PR (2006) Responsive parenting: establishing early foundations for social, communication, and independent problem-solving skills. Developmental Psychology 42(4): 627-642

257. Meins E (1997) Security of attachment and the social development of cognition. Psychology Press/Erlbaum (UK) Taylor & Francis, Hove, UK

258. Meins E et al (2001) Rethinking maternal sensitivity: mothers' comments on infants' mental processes predict security of attachment at 12 months. The Journal of Child Psychology and Psychiatry and Allied Disciplines 42(5): 637-648

259. Lindquist KA, MacCormack JK, Shablack H (2015) The role of language in emotion: predictions from psychological constructionism. Frontiers in Psychology 6: 444

260. Cantor P et al (2019) Malleability, plasticity, and individuality: how children learn and develop in context. Applied Developmental Science 24(3): 307-337

261. Luo Y, Baillargeon R (2005) When the ordinary seems unexpected: evidence for incremental physical knowledge in young infants. Cognition 95(3): 297-328

262. Stahl AE, Feigenson L (2015) Observing the unexpected enhances infants' learning and exploration. Science 348(6230): 91-94

263. Hespos SJ et al (2016) Five-month-old infants have general knowledge of how nonsolid substances behave and interact. Psychological Science 27(2): 244-256

264. Knickmeyer RC et al (2008) A structural MRI study of human brain development from birth to 2 years. The Journal of Neuroscience 28(47): 12176-12182

265. Bhardwaj RD et al (2006) Neocortical neurogenesis in humans is restricted to development. Proceedings of the National Academy of Sciences 103(33): 12564-12568

266. Rakic P (2006) No more cortical neurons for you. Science 313(5789): 928-929

267. Nowakowski RS (2006) Stable neuron numbers from cradle to grave. Proceedings of the National Academy of Sciences 103(33): 12219-12220

268. Christakis DA et al (2018) How early media exposure may affect cognitive function: a review of results from observations in humans and experiments in mice. Proceedings of the National Academy of Sciences 115(40): 9851-9858

269. Dawson G, Ashman S, Carver L (2000) The role of early experience in shaping behavioral and brain development and its implications for social policy. Development and Psychopathology 12: 695-712

270. Bernier A, Calkins SD, Bell MA (2016) Longitudinal associations between the quality of mother-infant interactions and brain development across infancy. Child Development 87(4): 1159-1174

271. Tierney AL, Nelson CA III (2009) Brain development and the role of experience in the early years. Zero Three 30(2): 9-13

272. Chechik G, Meilijson I, Ruppin E (1998) Synaptic pruning in development: a computational account. Neural Computation 10: 1759-1777

273. Gopnik A (2010) The philosophical baby: what children's minds tell us about truth, love, and the meaning of life. Picador, New York, NY, USA

274. Bruer JT (1998) The brain and child development: time for some critical thinking. Public Health Reports 113(5): 388-397

275. Wastell D, White S (2012) Blinded by neuroscience: social policy, the family and the infant brain. Families, Relationships and Societies 1(3): 397-414

276. Messer DJ (2002) Mastery motivation: an introduction to theories and issues. Pp 13-28 in: Mastery motivation in early childhood (ed Messer DJ). Routledge, London, UK

277. Bambach S et al (2016) Objects in the center: how the infant's body constrains infant scenes. Pp 132-137 in: Proceedings of the Joint IEEE International Conference on Development and Learning and Epigenetic Robotics

278. Adolph KE, Joh AS (2007) Motor development: how infants get into the act. Pp 63-80 in: Introduction to infant development (ed Slater A, Lewis M), Oxford University Press, New York, NY, USA

279. Pin T, Eldridge B, Galea MP (2007) A review of the effects of sleep position, play position, and equipment use on motor development in infants. Developmental Medicine and Child Neurology 49(11): 858-867

280. Visser MM, Franzsen D (2010) The association of an omitted crawling milestone with pencil grasp and control in five- and six-year-old children. South African Journal of Occupational Therapy 40: 19-23

281. Bell MA, Fox NA (1996) Crawling experience is related to changes in cortical organization during infancy: evidence from EEG coherence. Developmental Psychobiology 29(7): 551-561

282. Gonzalez SL, Reeb-Sutherland BC, Nelson EL (2016) Quantifying motor experience in the infant brain: EEG power, coherence, and mu desynchronization. Frontiers in Psychology 7: 216

283. Connell G, McCarthy C (2013) A moving child Is a learning child: how the body teaches the brain to think (birth to Age 7). Free Spirit Publishing, Minneapolis, MN, USA

284. Abbott A, Bartlett D (2001) Infant motor development and equipment use in the home. Child: Care, Health and Development 27(3): 295-306

285. Yogman M et al (2018) The power of play: a pediatric role in enhancing development in young children. Pediatrics 142(3): e20182058

286. Rubin K (1977) Play behaviors of young children. Young children 32(6): 16-24

287. Parten MB (1932) Social participation among pre-school children. The Journal of Abnormal and Social Psychology 27(3): 243-269

288. Adolph KE, Hoch JE (2019) Motor development: embodied, embedded, enculturated, and enabling. Annual Review of Psychology 70: 141-164

289. Adolph KE et al (2012) How do you learn to walk? Thousands of steps and dozens of falls per day. Psychological science 23(11): 1387-1394

290. Alexander GM, Wilcox T, Woods R (2009) Sex differences in infants' visual interest in toys. Archives of Sexual Behavior 38(3): 427-433

291. Todd BK, Barry JA, Thommessen SA (2017) Preferences for 'gender-typed' toys in boys and girls aged 9 to 32 months. Infant and Child Development 26(3): e1986

292. Zimmerman FJ, Christakis DA, Meltzoff AN (2007) Television and DVD/video viewing in children younger than 2 years. Archives of Pediatrics and Adolescent Medicine 161(5): 473-479

293. Vandewater EA et al (2007) Digital childhood: electronic media and technology use among infants, toddlers, and preschoolers. Pediatrics 119(5): e1006-e1015

294. Anderson DR, Pempek TA (2005) Television and very young children. American Behavioral Scientist 48(5): 505-522

295. Anderson DR, Hanson KG (2010) From blooming, buzzing confusion to media literacy: the early development of television viewing. Developmental Review 30(2): 239-255

296. Thompson DA, Christakis DA (2005) The association between television viewing and irregular sleep schedules among children less than 3 years of age. Pediatrics 116(4): 851-856

297. Dawson D, Encel N (1993) Melatonin and sleep in humans. Journal of Pineal Research 15(1): 1-12

298. Posner MI, Rothbart MK, Voelker P (2016) Developing brain networks of attention. Current Opinion in Pediatrics 28(6): 720-724

299. Christakis DA et al (2004) Early television exposure and subsequent attentional problems in children. Pediatrics 113(4): 708-713

300. Haughton C, Aiken M, Cheevers C (2015) Cyber babies: the impact of emerging technology on the developing infant. Psychology 5(9): 504-518

301. Rideout VJ, Vandewater EA, Wartella EA (2003) Zero to six: Electronic media in the lives of infants, toddlers and preschoolers. The Henry J. Kaiser Family Foundation report: https://www.kff.org/wp-content/uploads/2013/01/zero-to-six-electronic-media-in-the-lives-of-infants-toddlers-and-preschoolers-pdf.pdf (accessed on June 22, 2021)

302. Hanson K (2017) The influence of early media exposure on children's development and learning. Doctoral Dissertation. University of Massachusetts Amherst, MA, USA

303. Schmidt ME et al (2008) The effects of background television on the toy play behavior of very young children. Child development 79(4): 1137-1151

304. Kuhl PK, Tsao F-M, Liu H-M (2003) Foreign-language experience in infancy: effects of short-term exposure and social interaction on phonetic learning. Proceedings of the National Academy of Sciences 100(15): 9096-9101

305. Doige N (2007) The brain that changes itself. Viking, New York, NY, USA

306. van Ijzendoorn MH et al (1998) Attunement between parents and professional caregivers: a comparison of childrearing attitudes in different child-care settings. Journal of Marriage and the Family 60: 771-781

307. The OECD Family Database (2019) The Organisation for Economic Co-operation and Development http://www.oecd.org/els/family/database.htm (accessed on June 22, 2021)

308. Johnson MH, Lloyd-Fox S (2008) Do we study what parents want us to? Developmental Science 11: iii-iv

309. NICHD Early Child Care Research Network (1997)The effects of infant child care on infant-mother attachment security: results of the NICHD Study of Early Child Care. Child development 68(5): 860-879

310. Vandell DL (2004) Early child care: the known and the unknown. Merrill-Palmer Quarterly 50(3): 387-414

311. Belsky J et al (2007) Are there long-term effects of early child care? Child Development 78(2): 681-701

312. Albers EM et al (2016) Cortisol levels of infants in center care across the first year of life: links with quality of care and infant temperament. Stress 19(1): 8-17

313. Watamura SE et al (2003) Morning-to-afternoon increases in cortisol concentrations for infants and toddlers at child care: age differences and behavioral correlates. Child Development 74(4): 1006-1020

314. Ahnert L et al (2004) Transition to child care: associations with infant—mother attachment, infant negative emotion, and cortisol elevations. Child Development 75(3): 639-650

315. Scher A et al (2010) Sleep quality, cortisol levels, and behavioral regulation in toddlers. Developmental Psychobiology 52(1): 44-53

316. Vermeer HJ et al (2016) Quality of child care using the environment rating scales: a meta-analysis of international studies. International Journal of Early Childhood 48(1): 33-60

317. D'Angiulli A, Schibli K (2016) How neuroendocrinology can contribute to early childhood education and care: cortisol as a supplementary indicator of quality. Prospects 46(2): 281-299

318. Van IJzendoorn MH, Sagi A, Lambermon MW (1992) The multiple caretaker paradox: data from Holland and Israel. New Directions for Child and Adolescent Development 1992(57): 5-24

319. Pessanha M et al (2017) Stability and change in teacher-infant interaction quality over time. Early Childhood Research Quarterly 40: 87-97

320. Elfer P, Page J (2015) Pedagogy with babies: perspectives of eight nursery managers. Early Child Development and Care 185(11-12): 1762-1782

321. Page J (2011) Do mothers want professional carers to love their babies? Journal of Early Childhood Research 9(3): 310-323

322. Recchia SL, Shin M, Snaider C (2018) Where is the love? Developing loving relationships as an essential component of professional infant care. International Journal of Early Years Education 26(2): 142-158

323. Bowlby R (2007) Babies and toddlers in non-parental daycare can avoid stress and anxiety if they develop a lasting secondary attachment bond with one carer who is consistently accessible to them. Attachment and Human Development 9(4): 307-319

324. Ebbeck M, Yim HYB (2009) Rethinking attachment: fostering positive relationships between infants, toddlers and their primary caregivers. Early Child Development and Care 179(7): 899-909

325. Daniel J, Shapiro J (1996) Infant transitions: home to center-based child care. Child and Youth Care Forum 25: 11-123

326. Chazan-Cohen R et al (2017) Working toward a definition of infant/toddler curricula: intentionally furthering the development of individual children within responsive relationships. Report #2017-15 prepared for the Office of Planning, Research and Evaluation, Administration for Children and Families

327. Pocovi N et al (2019) Analysis of infant physical activity in the childcare environment: an observational study. Infant Behavior and Development 57: 101338

328. Solomon R, Martin K, Cottington E (1993) Spoiling an infant: further support for the construct. Topics in Early Childhood Special Education 13(2): 175-183

329. Mintz S (2004) Huck's raft: a history of American childhood. Harvard University Press, Cambridge, MA, USA

330. Gerber M (1998) Dear parent: caring for infants with respect. Resources for Infant Educarers, Los Angeles, CA, USA

331. Lansbury J (2014) Elevating child care: a guide to respectful parenting. JLML Press, Malibu, CA, USA

332. Fisher AV, Godwin KE, Seltman H (2014) Visual environment, attention allocation, and learning in young children: when too much of a good thing may be bad. Psychological science 25(7): 1362-1370

333. Dauch C et al (2018) The influence of the number of toys in the environment on toddlers' play. Infant Behavior and Development 50: 78-87

334. Hymes JL (1994) The child under 6. Consortium Publishing

335. Davis L, Keyser J (2012) Becoming the parent you want to be: a sourcebook of strategies for the first five years. Harmony, New York, NY, USA

336. Tamis-LeMonda CS, Kuchirko Y, Song L (2014) Why is infant language learning facilitated by parental responsiveness? Current Directions in Psychological Science 23(2): 121-126

337. Fitzpatrick EM et al (2014) How HANDy are baby signs? A systematic review of the impact of gestural communication on typically developing, hearing infants under the age of 36 months. First Language 34(6): 486-509

338. Trehub SE (2016) Infant musicality. Pp 387-398 in: The Oxford handbook of music psychology (ed Hallam S, Cross I, Thaut MH). Oxford University Press, New York, NY, USA

339. Rosenkoetter S, Barton L (2002) Bridges to literacy: early routines that promote later school success. Zero to Three 22(4): 33-38

340. Underdown A et al (2006) Massage intervention for promoting mental and physical health in infants aged under six months. Cochrane Database of Systematic Reviews 4: CD005038

341. Gerber M, Johnson A (1998) Your self-confident baby: how to encourage your child's natural abilities from the very start. John Wiley and Sons, New York, NY, USA

342. Faircloth C, Hoffman DM, Layne LL (2013) Parenting in global perspective: negotiating ideologies of kinship, self and politics. Routledge, London, UK

343. Swain JE et al (2007) Brain basis of early parent—infant interactions: psychology, physiology, and in vivo functional neuroimaging studies. Journal of Child Psychology and Psychiatry 48(3-4): 262-287

344. Swain JE et al (2014) Approaching the biology of human parental attachment: brain imaging, oxytocin and coordinated assessments of mothers and fathers. Brain Research 1580: 78-101

345. Gustafsson E et al (2013) Fathers are just as good as mothers at recognizing the cries of their baby. Nature communications 4(1): 1-6

346. Abraham E et al (2014) Father's brain is sensitive to childcare experiences. Proceedings of the National Academy of Sciences 111(27): 9792-9797

347. Young KS et al (2016) Evidence for a caregiving instinct: rapid differentiation of infant from adult vocalizations using magnetoencephalography. Cerebral Cortex 26(3): 1309-1321

348. Schaller M (2018) The parental care motivational system and why it matters (for everyone). Current Directions in Psychological Science 27(5): 295-301

349. Bornstein MH et al (2010) Parenting knowledge: experiential and sociodemographic factors in European American mothers of young children. Developmental Psychology 46(6): 1677-1693

350. Zero to Three (2016) Tuning in: parents of young children speak up about what they think, know and need. National Parent Survey Report. https://www.zerotothree.org/resources/1425-national-parent-survey-report (accessed on June 24, 2021)

351. Papoušek H, Papoušek M (2002) Intuitive parenting. PP 183-203 in: Handbook of Parenting. Biology and Ecology of Parenting (ed Bornstein MH). Lawrence Erlbaum Associates Publishers, Mahwah, NJ, USA

352. Hodgkinson GP, Langan-Fox J, Sadler-Smith E (2008) Intuition: a fundamental bridging construct in the behavioural sciences. British Journal of Psychology 99(1): 1-27

353. Baylor AL (1997) A three-component conception of intuition: immediacy, sensing relationships, and reason. New Ideas in Psychology 15(2): 185-194

354. Myers DG, Myers DG (2002) Intuition: its powers and perils. Yale University Press, New Haven, CT, USA

355. Koester LS, Lahti-Harper E (2010) Mother-infant hearing status and intuitive parenting behaviors during the first 18 months. American Annals of the Deaf 155(1): 5-18

356. Bornstein MH (2012) Cultural approaches to parenting. Parenting: Science and Practice 12: 212-221

357. Morelli GA, Rothbaum F (2007) Situating the child in context: attachment relationships and self-regulation in different cultures. Pp 500-527 in: Handbook of cultural psychology (eds Kitayama S, Cohen D) The Guilford Press, New York, NY, USA

358. Bornstein MH (2015) Culture, parenting, and zero-to-threes. Zero to Three 35(4): 2-9

359. Bronson P, Merryman A (2009) NurtureShock: new thinking about children. Twelve, New York, NY, USA

360. Lufityanto G, Donkin C, Pearson J (2016) Measuring intuition: nonconscious emotional information boosts decision accuracy and confidence. Psychological Science 27(5): 622-634

361. Sayer LC, Bianchi SM, Robinsn JP (2019) Are parents investing less in children? Trends in mothers' and fathers' time with children. American Journal of Sociology 110(1): 1-43

362. Gauthier AH, Smeedeng TM, Furstenberg FF (2004) Are parents investing less time in children? Trends in selected industrialized countries. Population and Development Review 30(4): 647-671

363. Dotti Sani GM, Treas J (2016) Educational gradients in parents' child-care time across countries, 1965-2012. Journal of Marriage and Family 78(4): 1083-1096

364. Ennis LR (2014) Intensive mothering: the cultural contradictions of modern motherhood. Demeter Press, Bradford, ON, Canada

365. Yavorsky JE, Dush CMK, Schoppe-Sullivan SJ (2015) The production of inequality: the gender division of labor across the transition to parenthood. Journal of Marriage and Family 77(3): 662-679

366. OECD (2018) Organization for Economic Cooperation and Development Family Database https://www.oecd.org/els/soc/PF2_1_Parental_leave_systems.pdf (accessed on June 24, 2021)

367. Twiggs JE, McQuillan J, Ferree MM (1999) Meaning and measurement: reconceptualizing measures of the division of household labor. Journal of Marriage and Family 61(3): 712-724

368. Craig L (2007) Is there really a second shift, and if so, who does it? A time-diary investigation. Feminist Review 86(1):149-170

369. Offer S, Schneider B (2011) Revisiting the gender gap in time-use patterns: multitasking and well-being among mothers and fathers in dual-earner families. American Sociological Review 76(6): 809-833

370. Spink A, Cole C, Waller M (2008) Multitasking behavior. Annual Review of Information Science and Technology 42(1): 93-118

371. Allen SM, Hawkins AJ (1999) Maternal gatekeeping: mothers' beliefs and behaviors that inhibit greater father involvement in family work. Journal of Marriage and Family 61(1): 199-212

372. Daminger A (2019) The cognitive dimension of household labor. American Sociological Review 84(4): 609-633

373. Fagan J, Barnett M (2003) The relationship between maternal gatekeeping, paternal competence, mothers' attitudes about the father role, and father involvement. Journal of Family Issues 24(8): 1020-1043

374. Schoppe-Sullivan SJ et al (2015) Who are the gatekeepers? Predictors of maternal gatekeeping. Parenting: Science and Practice 15(3): 166-186

375. Schoppe-Sullivan SJ, Fagan J (2020) The evolution of fathering research in the 21st century: persistent challenges, new directions. Journal of Marriage and Family 82(1): 175-197

376. Berry B. (2020) Motherwhelmed: challenging norms, untangling truths, and restoring our worth to the world. Revolution from Home, USA

377. Boddy AM et al (2015) Fetal microchimerism and maternal health: a review and evolutionary analysis of cooperation and conflict beyond the womb. Bioessays 37(10): 1106-1118

378. Ruppanner L, Brandén M, Turunen J (2017) Does unequal housework lead to divorce? Evidence from Sweden. Sociology 52(1): 75-94

379. Wetherbee K (2012) Joy, or "Just Wait?" (Diving for Pearls blog article) https://katiewetherbee.com/2012/02/06/joy-or-just-wait/?tag=powofmom-20 (accessed on June 24, 2021)

INDEX

Made in the USA
Las Vegas, NV
24 September 2022

55879119R00179